the
HOLISTIC
HEALTH
handbook

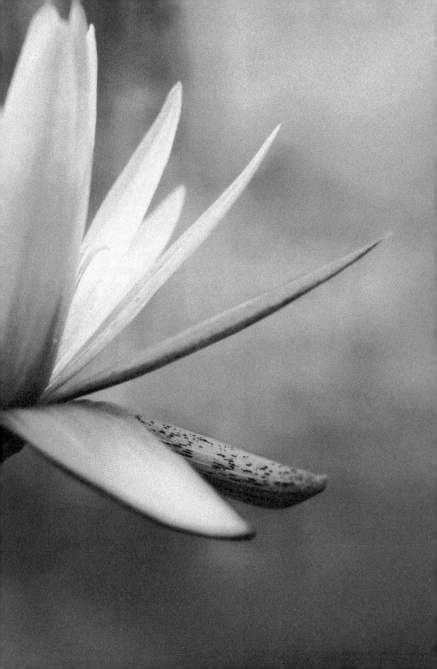

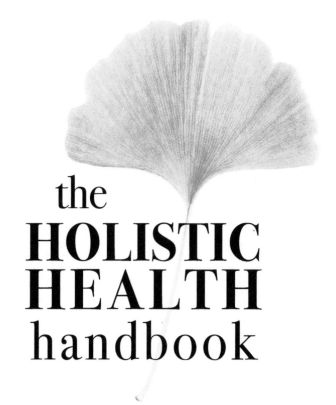

the
HOLISTIC
HEALTH
handbook

HEALING REMEDIES *for* COMMON AILMENTS

Kim Lam, AADP, CHHC

ROCKRIDGE
PRESS

For general information on our other products and services or to obtain technical support, please contact our Customer Care Department within the United States at (866) 744-2665, or outside the United States at (510) 253-0500.

Rockridge Press publishes its books in a variety of electronic and print formats. Some content that appears in print may not be available in electronic books, and vice versa.

Interior and Cover Designer: Regina Stadnik
Art Producer: Sue Bischofberger
Editor: Andrea Leptinsky
Production Editor: Emily Sheehan

Photography © ddukang/iStock, cover and pp. iii, v, 23, and 77; LordRunar /iStock, p. ii; Helene Dujardin, pp. v, 57, and 58; Abby Mortenson/Stocksy, p. 2-3; Eileen Kumpf/shutterstock, pp. 4, 8, 26, 40, 50, 62, and 70; Almaje/iStock, p. 57; Arundhati Sathe /iStock, p. 58; and Lucia Loiso, p. 78-79
Illustration © GreyLilac/shutterstock (gingko pattern throughout).

ISBN: Print 978-1-64739-608-4 | eBook 978-1-64739-609-1

R0

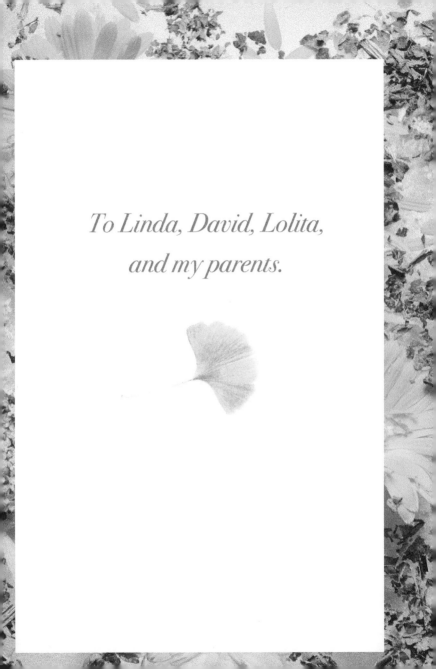

To Linda, David, Lolita,

and my parents.

CONTENTS

INTRODUCTION

In 2012, I was lying on the bathroom floor clutching my stomach and screaming in pain. My stress levels were at a peak from working a fast-paced corporate pharmaceutical sales job. My sleep was erratic, and stomach pains haunted me weekly.

After numerous doctor visits and testing, I was left with no answers, and I was given a pill to ease the stomach pain. My health was declining, and I didn't know how or where to go to fix it. It turns out I was suffering from Irritable Bowel Syndrome (IBS), adrenal fatigue, stubborn weight gain, and insulin resistance.

After the diagnosis, I took a course on holistic nutrition that opened my eyes to how you can heal your body from common ailments with certain foods. I learned about holistic medicine and how important it is to treat the body as a whole system. This marked the beginning of my journey into holistic healing and my commitment to spread awareness about this healing approach.

I learned to be my own health advocate and seek alternative practitioners for treatment. I learned to manage my stress using meditation, essential oils, and exercise. I also began paying attention to the role of nutrition and how it affected my health. I ate more whole foods, took herbal concoctions and supplements like probiotics that alleviated my IBS, and spent a lot of time gardening and hiking. I was so excited about my own healing journey that I decided to commit to teaching and spreading awareness about this approach to healing.

A few years after supporting local clients with similar health issues, I applied the same principles of holistic health to my toddler's eczema. At one point he was getting sick every other week, suffering from stomach problems, and getting visible rashes on his face, arms, and legs. We were given a round of antibiotics each time we visited the pediatrician's office, but I had a feeling they weren't needed. It turns out he had a food intolerance to dairy, eggs, and gluten, which was causing the issues. After getting to the root cause of his problems and using a holistic treatment approach, today he is a happier kid, most of the eczema issues have subsided, and his immune system has improved. I am confident that by applying holistic medicine such as essential oils, alternative supplements, and herbs, he is now on a productive healing path.

I am grateful for the many benefits of holistic medicine, and it is my mission to bring this powerful tool to you so you can be empowered to find your own healing path. You can feel good and thrive! My wish is to help make this practice more accessible to more people. It is important to see the patient as a whole and to provide holistic care and treatment, instead of just viewing the patient through the lens of their diagnoses.

In this book, I'll show you the wisdom behind holistic healing, why it's important, and how to incorporate the practices into your daily life. Be open-minded and don't feel like you have to know everything right away or apply all the practices in order to achieve results.

A central feature of this book is that it offers remedies for common, everyday ailments that are meant to provide relief and help alleviate symptoms. This book is not meant to replace your doctor's medical recommendations, nor is it meant to treat or cure any illness. If you are currently suffering from serious health issues, please work with your health-care providers before embarking on any new healing regimen.

Getting the Most Out of This Book

This book is meant to be a guide; think of it as a tool kit of useful remedies at your fingertips. We'll start with an introduction to the history of holistic health and how it has come to be more accepted in society today, and then discuss various holistic practices and how to integrate them into your daily life.

The book is presented in three parts. Part 1 introduces holistic health and why you should consider integrating these healing modalities into your health treatment plan. We will discuss the six critical aspects of a balanced body: environment, digestion, sleep, exercise, passion, and nutrition. Successful holistic healing requires that you strive for balance in each of these areas in your life.

Part 2 will highlight various holistic practices that are most commonly used today. This section will be helpful to understand what remedies are available and how you can apply them to your healing journey. You will learn about effective alternative practices for the most common, everyday health issues.

Then, in part 3, you'll learn how to put some of these remedies into practice. You'll be given a holistic tool kit that provides three different remedies for each of the ailments covered. Most of these remedies will be very easy to make or execute. Many require ingredients derived from nature or simply from your kitchen cabinet.

No matter where you are in your healing journey, the remedies found in this book can help support your goal to achieve more balance in your body. If you're here to feel empowered and to take control of your own healing journey, this book is for you.

PART 1

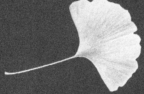

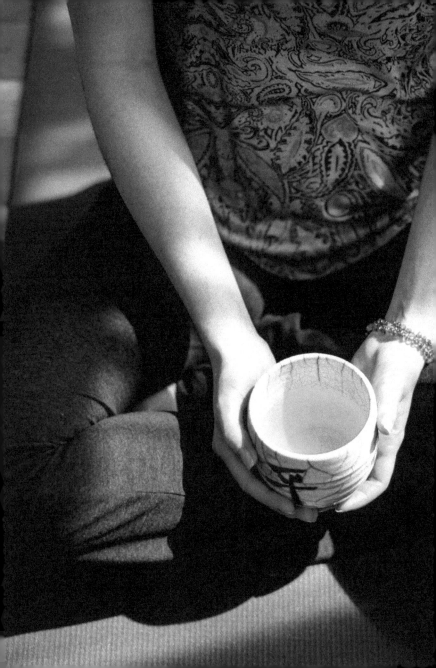

Understanding Holistic Health

In medicine, "holism" refers to managing the *person* as a whole, not just the symptoms or disease. Holistic healing requires the integration of mind, body, and spirit to maintain and restore balance in the body. It also emphasizes the importance of the whole body and the interdependence of its parts. A perfect analogy would be to think of the body as an orchestra, where each part is one instrument; the whole orchestra sounds much better when each part is in harmony with one another.

CHAPTER 1

The Tradition of Holistic Healing

Holistic healing was the foundation of ancient health care thousands of years ago. Today, holistic health practitioners believe that healing is most effective when you take into consideration the whole body rather than focusing on just the illness and symptoms. The holistic approach is about honoring the mind-body connection and treating the whole person using a variety of clinically proven techniques.

The Ancient System of Health: Mind, Body, and Spirit

In 400 BCE, Hippocrates, the father of medicine, stressed the healing power of nature in his school of medicine. His philosophy was not to focus on the disease but instead to study the whole patient, including their emotional state of mind, their environment, and also their spiritual beliefs. He was a proponent of self-healing. Socrates, a Greek philosopher and the founder of Western philosophy, also emphasized the value of thinking holistically and that our health was our responsibility.

Other physicians at the time were more focused on actively eradicating the patient's illness. The two different approaches of healing were debated for centuries until the discovery of germs. Hippocrates's teachings and philosophy came to an end upon the discovery of germs, which began the practice of focused intervention. Since most diseases could be treated by drugs such as penicillin, physicians began focusing on developing medicines to manage and treat symptoms, which is the main goal of conventional medicine today. The holistic view of the patient, Hippocrates's view, took a back seat.

This modern approach to healing caused a disconnect between the patient and their body's natural, innate ability to heal. The focused intervention approach, in addition to modern lifestyle factors such as poor diet, inactivity, and chronic stress, would eventually expose the pitfalls of conventional medicine. Physicians paid less attention to recommending healthy lifestyle choices, emphasizing the importance of emotional health, and acknowledging environmental factors. Instead the main focus was on treating the patient's symptoms with medication. Many physicians dispensed with what they considered outdated treatments such as herbalism and Traditional Chinese Medicine (TCM).

Eventually, it became apparent that there are limitations to the approach of treating the symptoms instead of the patient as a whole. Not every disease was responding in favor of the scientific treatment. Sadly, some of these scientific approaches were causing more harm to the patient than the disease itself.

In time, people began to seek alternative forms of medicine. This led to a renewed interest in holistic healing in the 1970s. Holistic health encompasses many modalities of treatment, including massage therapy, acupuncture, meditation, homeopathy, and Reiki energy healing. Many core practices and principles of alternative medicine are based on the paradigms of traditional Chinese philosophy. Traditional Chinese Medicine is based on Taoist principles and is still widely used throughout Asia today.

This brief history of medicine shows that many of the practices used today have been around for thousands of years. The practice of using alternative medicine to deal with common health issues is rising in popularity, and it's my hope that more people will discover and use these helpful practices.

The Five Aspects of Holistic Health

Emotional | Mental | Physical | Spiritual | Social

Holistic health means looking beyond the physical body to address emotional, mental, physical, spiritual, and social health. Collectively, these five aspects enable a person to fully live each day in the healthiest, happiest way possible. If one area is compromised, most likely other areas will be as well. Recall the analogy of the body as an orchestra; each of these five aspects must work together in order for a body to function optimally.

CHAPTER 2

Finding Your Balance with Holistic Healing

Hippocrates said it best: "Nature itself is the best physician." He advocated for nature's ability to heal illness and restore health and vitality to humans. When you live with balance and embrace the healing power of plants as food and medicine, you can achieve holistic health.

The Dimensions of Holistic Healing

Your body wants to be healed. One of the most powerful discoveries that you'll make is that your body is not designed to get sick, and when it does, it does its best to repair itself. In order for holistic healing to be successful, it is important that you strive for a well-coordinated balance in all aspects of your life. Let's take a look at the six essential aspects of balance.

1. ENVIRONMENT

Ailments that are commonly associated with an imbalance in this area include depression, insomnia, and chronic stress.

Humans follow a circadian rhythm, which is a sleep-wake pattern governed by the 24-hour day-night cycle. Circadian rhythms are physical, mental, and behavioral changes in living beings that adhere to this cycle. When we are disconnected from this natural rhythm, our sleep quality and overall health can be negatively affected.

In our modern world, we spend much of our time indoors exposed to artificial light, which puts us out of sync with natural circadian rhythms. Several studies show that rooms with bright artificial light can negatively affect your health. Staying up late staring at a brightly lit computer or phone screen can increase your risk for obesity, depression, insomnia, diabetes, and more.

If we live in tune with our natural biological clocks and circadian rhythms, we will be more energized and awake in the morning and wind down more easily in the evening. Our bodies naturally follow the sunset and sunrise; we wake up to the light of the sun and begin to wind down when the sun sets. We have a primal need for sunlight and fresh air.

For example, our bodies produce a natural hormone called melatonin, which not only helps us sleep but also boosts the immune system, lowers cholesterol, and supports the functions of other organs. Artificial light suppresses the production of this hormone. Natural light is best; in fact, many studies show evidence that spending even a few minutes in sunlight can significantly reduce stress and have a complex, positive impact on emotions.

2. DIGESTION

Ailments that are commonly associated with an imbalance in this area include chronic constipation, allergies, and skin issues such as eczema.

Digestion breaks down the foods you eat into nutrients, which the body uses for energy, growth, and repair. If your body cannot properly digest and absorb nutrients and eliminate waste products, it is hard to achieve optimal wellness. Over time, digestive problems can cause chronic illness. Chronic digestive problems can also cause inflammation and have an array of negative effects on the rest of the body including the skin, immune system, and brain.

It is imperative that you have a properly functioning digestive system since it also acts as a communication center to and from the brain. This is the reason many experts now refer to our gut as the "second brain." Interestingly, our gut and brain also play a role in our stress levels, mood, and state of mind. For example, the gut produces more than 90 percent of the body's serotonin, a hormone that helps regulate our mood and emotions.

On the other hand, stress can cause digestive issues like bloating and nausea and can trigger symptoms in people who have irritable bowel syndrome or other gastrointestinal conditions. Heeding the signals of your gut and increasing your awareness of the nutritional and digestive properties of food can help you become more attuned to your own unique digestive health.

3. EXERCISE

Ailments that are commonly associated with an imbalance in this area include depression, osteoporosis, obesity, and stress.

The body is designed to move and not be stagnant. When you start moving on a daily basis, you will not only see the tangible results of a strong and sculpted body, but you will also optimize the flow of energy throughout your body.

For example, the lymphatic system does not have an organ to move lymph throughout the body like the heart pumps blood throughout the body. Because of this, the lymphatic system relies on movement of the muscles and joints to pump lymph throughout the body. When you stop moving, this energy becomes stagnant, and illness can occur. Since the body is connected to the mind, your mind can suffer as well. When the flow of energy between the emotional, mental, and physical aspects of your being is interrupted, it creates an imbalance that could result in disease.

Exercise, or any form of movement, is essential to an individual's overall health. It benefits not only our physical bodies but also our mental and emotional well-being. One side benefit of exercise is that it can trigger your body to release endorphins (often referred to as "feel-good hormones"), giving you a sense of happiness or even euphoria. Try to recall the last time you danced at a party and felt free and exhilarated; this is a perfect example of how your body's movement can affect your mind.

4. NUTRITION

Ailments that are commonly caused by an imbalance in this area include digestive disorders, thyroid imbalance, high blood pressure, heart disease, hormone imbalance, and diabetes.

What we eat greatly influences our health. Most Western cultures today produce an abundance of easily available food. Compared with the days of famine and starvation, this is, of course, a good thing. However, in the United States, this abundance has led to some significant health risks.

As a nation we are overeating, but at the same time, we are undernourished. We're also eating more ultra-processed foods that have been altered from their natural form such as flavored potato chips, candy bars, and soda. Faced with an abundant array of modern food products, people are naturally tempted by convenience. Most people would prefer not to worry about how their food is processed or what it contains, but there are many problems with highly processed food, including the additions of excess sugar, preservatives, dyes, and unhealthy fats.

In addition, nutrients, vitamins, minerals, and fiber—all of which serve important roles in maintaining good health—can be destroyed when food is processed. For example, when the outer layers of fruits, vegetables, and whole grains are peeled away, plant nutrients (called phytochemicals or phytonutrients) can also be removed. This is problematic because these nutrients can keep you healthy and prevent disease.

Highly processed foods are also associated with the obesity epidemic and rising prevalence of chronic diseases like heart disease and diabetes. Whole foods—foods that have not been processed and remain in their natural state—are not associated with any of these health issues. And, in fact, many whole foods are beneficial for your health. For example, fruits, vegetables, whole grains, legumes, and nuts contain fiber, which is essential for balancing blood sugar, improving digestion and regularity, and helping you feel satiated.

When you eat clean whole foods that are minimally processed, true health becomes a possibility. My goal is to turn this possibility into reality. Your goal should be to upgrade the quality of your food with every bite. Whatever your diet preference is—paleo, vegetarian, vegan—try to eat as many whole foods as you can.

5. PASSION

Ailments that are commonly associated with an imbalance in this area include depression, heart disease, Alzheimer's, a weakened immune system, and anxiety.

Passion is a powerful healing tool. Think of it as a source of unlimited energy from your own soul. Studies show that pursuing your passions can improve your physical health and physiological well-being.

Think about all the things that are stimulating for you, whether it's dancing, listening to music, collecting art, cooking, spending time outdoors, or sipping coffee over a deep, meaningful conversation with a friend. We are naturally social beings and crave meaningful relationships with others. Being loved, being understood, and being connected to others can have a profound effect on your health.

Whatever it is that you love and enjoy doing, whatever is important and meaningful to you, try to do that activity every day. When you engage in activities that you are passionate about, you experience increased happiness. There is a direct correlation between happiness and good health, resulting in improved mental health, lower blood pressure, and lower risk of stress, anxiety, and depression.

In addition, having a passion can provide you with a drive for self-improvement and purpose. Many people also find that pursuing their passion has led them to discover their life's purpose, as well as provided them with the clarity, fuel, motivation, and confidence to step outside their comfort zone.

6. SLEEP

Ailments that are commonly associated with an imbalance in this area include poor thyroid function, hormonal imbalance, obesity, a weakened immune system, and anxiety.

Let's be honest—most of us aren't getting enough sleep. And if we are, perhaps it's not a quality of sleep that can promote health. The National Sleep Foundation suggests that on average adults need about seven to nine hours of sleep per night. You may wonder what this has to do with your overall health and vitality. You already know that a good night's sleep leaves you feeling rested and rejuvenated, but did you know that your body is also doing some important work while you sleep? For example, major restorative functions such as protein synthesis (the process by which cells make protein) and the liver's detoxification process (in which the liver cleanses the body of toxins and produces bile for healthy digestion) occur mostly during sleep.

Additionally, it's been well documented that adequate sleep can positively affect certain hormone levels in your body such as leptin, which decreases appetite, and ghrelin, which increases appetite. Also, lack of sleep causes your body to produce excess cortisol, a hormone that tends to contribute to increased stress and weight gain.

Now that you know about the major impact that sleep has on your overall wellness and your body's ability to heal, I hope you will choose to prioritize your sleep! Think of sleep as a free health tool that can help you improve your metabolism and immune system, lose weight, repair cells, detoxify, delay aging, increase cognitive function, and provide more energy.

Making Holistic Therapy Your Own

After reading about the potential benefits of holistic healing, I hope you're ready to dive right in. But before you do, let's take a moment to consider two central issues.

First, it's important to understand the meaning of the terms "safe" and "effective," which are often used to describe all kinds of health-care treatments, supplements, and devices. So, what do they mean? "Safe" generally means that the holistic therapy will not cause harm or be detrimental to your health. "Effective" means that the holistic therapy works in the way that it is intended to. The question to consider is what a claim of safety or effectiveness is based on. With conventional medicine, most treatments are scientifically tested through trials and research, and claims of safety and effectiveness are based on that. With holistic treatments, some scientific studies have been conducted, but generally, claims of safety and effectiveness are based on thousands of years of accumulated wisdom and experience. Keep in mind that our bodies are all different, so not all therapies—be they conventional or holistic—will work for all people.

Second, it's important to develop a plan for your own healing journey. Holistic health is about empowerment and personal responsibility. It is the sum of all your choices and actions that you take every single day; that means you harness the power within yourself to achieve lasting health and happiness. I encourage you to create a treatment plan that makes sense to you, but be sure to get your doctor's approval first. I am not suggesting that you abandon conventional medicine for complementary therapy or holistic practices, but I do believe that in many cases it could be to your benefit to incorporate holistic practices into your current treatment regimen. They can complement conventional care and be the key to successful outcomes. Let's take a look at how this might work:

You go to your doctor's office complaining of digestion problems, particularly constipation. She prescribes a laxative. You explain to her that you've had this problem before and the laxative only works temporarily. Then you ask her if she'd be okay with you visiting a naturopathic doctor, who you think could help you get to the root cause of the constipation. (Remember, holistic medicine aims to treat the root cause of an issue, and with constipation, a laxative would simply allow the patient to relieve themselves temporarily, not correct what's causing the constipation in the first place.)

Since health issues are different for everyone, a holistic treatment plan needs to be individualized. For some, it could be simple and straightforward. For others, it may take more time and trials. For more complex cases, you have to really understand and listen to what your body is trying to tell you. Be mindful that there is no such thing as a quick fix when it comes to healing. Have patience with where you are in your journey. Everyone heals at a different rate based upon their makeup and the nature of their ailment.

What is most critical to understand is that illness does not show up in one day. It is a collective of symptoms and signs that your body gives to you on a continual basis. So, when we try to heal, we must remember that it is not a linear process. True holistic healing should result in an improvement in all aspects of your life.

THREE QUESTIONS TO ASK BEFORE STARTING A HOLISTIC TREATMENT PLAN

Before you commit to any holistic treatment plan, you should ask yourself the following questions:

1. WHAT ARE THE RISKS?

Just because an herb or food is "natural" doesn't mean that it's safe. For example, some mushrooms are considered adaptogens—non-toxic plants that can be helpful in managing stress. However, not every species of wild mushroom is safe to eat. In addition, some therapies can also put you at risk if they interfere with a treatment or medication that you are currently receiving. These risks depend on each individual product or practice.

2. WHAT ARE THE POTENTIAL BENEFITS?

What will the holistic remedy do? Will it work? How will it contribute to my overall health? Find out what the holistic treatments will actually do for your ailment. How effective is the holistic remedy? Some remedies may help to relieve more than one symptom. For example, stress-reducing techniques may help reduce or prevent multiple ailments since chronic stress can be a root cause of many health symptoms. You must also keep in mind that your body is unique. Each person will respond to remedies in a different way.

3. WHAT IS THE EVIDENCE?

How much scientific evidence is there that the remedy is safe and effective? You can now find a large compilation of research studies on the National Center for Complementary and Integrative Health's website. Keep in mind that these scientific studies are relatively new and more are emerging each day. Always consider the source of these studies. Statements may be biased if they come from a specific company or promoter.

Although scientifically conducted studies are usually given more weight than anecdotes and stories, there is a gray area between objective evidence and the experience from ancient times. We must not ignore the accumulated wisdom of over 5,000 years. Always beware of claims that a particular treatment will be a quick fix or a miracle cure. If it sounds too good to be true, it probably is.

Conventional vs. Holistic Health Care

The term "holistic medicine" comes from the Greek word *halo*, which means "whole," and refers to the practice of medicine that treats the mind, body, and spirit. Holistic medicine differs from conventional Western medicine in terms of its philosophy and treatment. Conventional Western medicine is focused on illness and symptoms. Holistic medicine is focused on the whole person and views health as being influenced by a person's individual beliefs and lifestyle.

Diagnosis in Western medicine involves linking the patient's symptoms to a known disease or dysfunction. Advanced diagnostic tools are used to diagnose the disease and follow its progress. Holistic practitioners, on the other hand, analyze physical, nutritional, environmental, emotional, spiritual, and lifestyle factors to diagnose and recommend treatment. They search for the underlying causes of disease. For example, patients who suffer from chronic back pain may be given recommendations to add acupuncture, aromatherapy, massage, and herbs to the current traditional treatment plan set forth by their conventional doctor.

Disease management also varies between the two systems. Holistic treatments might include dietary changes, movement, meditation, guided imagery, massage therapy, acupuncture, and the use of herbs, all of which aim to bring balance back to the mind, body, and spirit. In Western medicine, treatment typically includes prescription medicine and sometimes physical therapy. The patient is not usually encouraged to make lifestyle and dietary changes.

PART 2

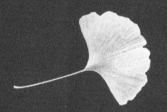

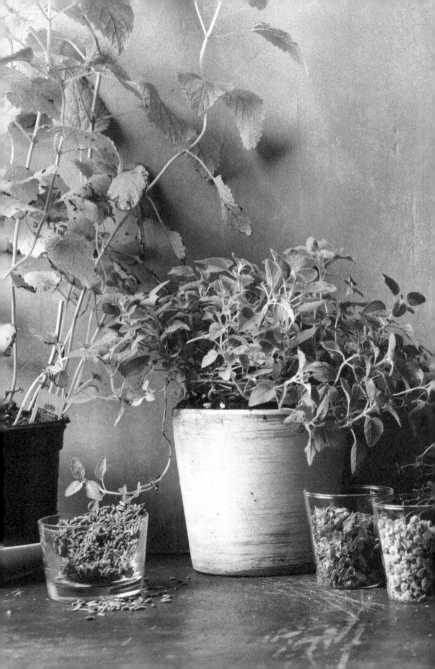

Healing Practices and Treatments

In this part I'll introduce you to various holistic healing practices and treatments. We will take a deep dive into the ones that are effective yet easy enough for you to explore on your own at home. They are designed to improve the body overall, with a focus on health. Treatments include alternative medical systems, food and supplements, herbal concoctions, exercise routines, stress relievers, and energy work. Note that this is not a comprehensive list of all available holistic healing practices but an introduction to some of the more common ones.

CHAPTER 3

Alternative Medical Systems

In this chapter we'll explore what are known as alternative medical systems, which comprise a group of practices and products that are generally not considered part of conventional medicine. Two of the most common of these systems are Traditional Chinese Medicine (TCM) and Ayurveda.

TCM and Ayurveda were developed in Eastern countries and have been used for centuries. Both systems of health care have one thing in common: they help facilitate restoration of balance in the body in a holistic way. These ancient practices can have positive and amazing effects.

Origins, Growth, and How They're Used Today

Alternative medical systems are built upon a broad, complete system of theories and practice. They have evolved independently over the years in different cultures.

TCM probably originated about 5,000 years ago, although the first recorded history goes back only about 2,000 years. Chinese legends claim that three emperors played a role in the history of TCM. TCM is based on the Chinese concept that disease results from disruption in the flow of *qi* (pronounced "chee"), or vital energy, through the body's pathways. This flow is the magic that regulates emotional, physical, mental, and spiritual balance and can be influenced by the opposite forces of energy known as yin and yang. TCM encompasses several practices that include the use of herbs and massage to help bring the body back to harmony and wellness. TCM also relies on the use of energy-based practices such as cupping and acupuncture; both are based on the belief that in order to maintain health, there must be an uninterrupted flow of energy throughout the 12 meridian pathways of the body, with each meridian corresponding to an organ.

Ayurveda means "the science of life" in Sanskrit. It originated in India more than 3,000 years ago and is still taught and practiced there today. Ayurveda's philosophy does not simply focus on the treatment of disease but on optimal well-being for the body, mind, and consciousness.

Ayurveda aims to balance the body's energy, which is made up of a combination of physical, mental, and emotional elements referred to as *vata*, *pitta*, and *kapha*. It is believed that health and wellness depend on a delicate balance of these three energies. Ayurveda treatments include diet, exercise, herbs, meditation, and controlled breathing. Ancient teachers also prescribe other practices to expand self-awareness such as meditation, cooking, eating fresh, seasonal whole foods, and adopting daily rituals.

There has been a significant increase in the practice of both TCM and Ayurveda over recent years. A study comparing TCM and Ayurveda found that China has been successful in introducing and promoting its therapies with more research and science-based approaches. In fact, there is a rapid increase in the number of licensed Chinese medicine providers in the United States.

There is also an increased demand for medicinal plants from India. Within the United States and European countries, botanical and herbal medicine use has grown. The World Health Organization has been actively creating strategies, guidelines, and standards for botanical medicine in response to the rise in their use. The *Herbal Medicinal Products Market: Global Industry Analysis (2012–2016) and Opportunity Assessment (2017–2027)* reports that the global market for herbal medicinal products is likely to reach $274 billion by 2027.

Both TCM and Ayurveda have remained popular in Eastern countries over the centuries, but they were virtually unknown in the West until the 1970s. Since then, their popularity has steadily grown. Despite the significant gains in health care and quality made possible through the innovative drugs and treatments created by the conventional medical industry, heart disease, prostate cancer, and other chronic diseases are still climbing each year. According to the Centers for Disease Control and Prevention, chronic disease accounts for about 75 percent of the nation's health-care spending. Hence, we're seeing an increased interest and need for alternative medical systems.

Today, although TCM has evolved into a complex diagnostic and treatment system, many of its original methods such as acupuncture, herbal remedies, cupping, and *gua sha* are still used today to alleviate a variety of ailments. For example, contemporary uses of TCM include the following:

- Acupuncture for certain pain or issues including lower back pain, neck pain, knee pain, carpal tunnel syndrome, muscle pain, headaches, migraines, fibromyalgia, and osteoporosis
- Ginger tea to alleviate nausea
- Tai chi to strengthen the immune system, increase flexibility, and decrease stress

- Cupping therapy for muscle pain and to aid in sports recovery

Contemporary uses of Ayurveda include the following:

- Meditation and controlled breathing for reducing stress
- Turmeric for reducing inflammation
- Massage with oils for reducing chronic pain and improving skin health

The increasing use of alternative therapies has been undertaken by some of the country's most respected hospitals, with doctors becoming more accepting of them as complementary treatments to conventional medicine. For example, gastroenterologist Dr. Linda Lee offers acupuncture and massage therapy at the Johns Hopkins Integrative Medicine & Digestive Center in Baltimore. The Osher Center for Integrative Medicine at the University of California, San Francisco, also offers a wide range of services including Chinese herbal medicine and Ayurveda.

Alternative medicine has played a huge role in the healing industry for centuries, and it's continuing to grow at a rapid rate today.

The Mind-Body-Spirit Connection

The integration of mind, body, and spirit is essential to holistic healing practices. This is based on the ancient theory that to have good health, you must have a positive spirit. You cannot ignore one aspect and expect the others to flourish.

TCM follows established diagnostic parameters for assessing the energy flow within the body and guiding it to a state of balance. It teaches that through this process, the body's organs will function as expected, positively affecting mind, body, and spirit. The benefits of TCM practices include reducing inflammation, improving muscle strength and flexibility, protecting cardiovascular health, and improving quality of sleep.

Acupuncture, for example, is one of the methods used in TCM to alleviate pain, but there's much more to it than that. When we feel pain, we must identify the imbalances that are causing the pain. Acupuncture helps pinpoint the pain source and restore balance to the energy forces in the body. As a result, the pain can diminish.

TCM can enhance mind-spirit harmony through specific nutrients, herbs, and acupressure. A balanced harmony associated with improved memory, cognitive skills, and stress relief can be achieved. For example, oolong tea can detoxify the brain and nourish the blood and spleen, while rosemary is a strong antioxidant that stimulates memory.

For many centuries, people have healed themselves through Ayurveda, which is India's traditional and time-proven method to establish physical, mental, and spiritual health. It is a way of living; a lifestyle that is medicinal. Ayurveda teaches us how to live in a healthy and fulfilling way and promotes heightened feelings of peace, happiness, bliss, and confidence. Ayurveda also teaches a lifestyle that prevents disease and optimizes health and well-being, focusing on the body, mind, and spirit instead of disease or symptoms. It reminds us that we are incredible self-healing machines and that we can regain (or maintain) optimal health by eating healing foods and living a healthy lifestyle.

Ayurveda teaches that when you are sick, your body is not broken. It is not failing you. It is simply out of balance, which means that it can be brought back into balance. With just a few lifestyle changes, your body can be strong enough to begin healing itself. This message can be very encouraging to people who suffer from chronic illnesses. Ayurveda also teaches physical strategies to improve digestion, practical ways to love yourself, and daily and seasonal routines to promote well-being. For example, deep pranayama is deep belly breathing that can promote digestion by stimulating metabolism. It's a simple breathing technique that you can practice at home.

Traditional Chinese Medicine and Holistic Health

Traditional Chinese Medicine (TCM) is a 5,000-year-old practice rooted in the ancient philosophy of Taoism. It has evolved into a complex diagnostic and treatment system, and many of its methods are still practiced today throughout the world, but especially in Asia.

There are a few key components of TCM.

TCM views the human body as a collective microcosm of the universe. We are interconnected with nature. Our minds, emotions, spirits, organs, and tissues all have distinct functions but are also interdependent. The body is viewed as a complex system powered by energy.

TCM is based on the concept that disease results from disruption in the flow of *qi* (pronounced "chee"), or vital energy, throughout the pathways of the body. That flow regulates emotional, physical, mental, and spiritual balance and can be influenced by the opposite forces of energy known as *yin* and *yang*. According to this theory, physical, emotional, and mental health problems can develop when the flow of qi is blocked or weakened.

TCM encompasses several practices including the use of herbs, massage, cupping, and acupuncture to bring the body back to harmony and balance. In order to be healthy, the body has to achieve this balanced state. TCM also focuses on strengthening the body's defense mechanism and enhances its ability to heal.

In summary, TCM teaches you how to live a well-balanced, harmonious life.

Acupressure, Healing Touch, and Massage

Acupressure therapy can be very effective in resolving many ailments that are by-products of daily living— particularly stress, headaches, and minor pain. It is similar to acupuncture except that, instead of using needles, it uses gentle manual pressure on specific points of the body to help clear blockages and restore energy flow. Pressure may be applied by hand or elbow. Originating from TCM, acupressure is based on the concept that energy flows along invisible pathways in the body called "meridians." Each meridian is connected to an organ. So, when the flow of energy gets blocked from stress, trauma, or injury, problems can arise.

Acupressure has also been found to be effective in easing nausea and vomiting. For example, a study that analyzed 22 clinical trials found that applying acupressure on the wrist decreased chemotherapy-induced nausea and vomiting. Acupressure can also help with muscular ailments like neck pain, soreness, lower back pain, and carpal tunnel syndrome. It can even help with constipation, migraines, and fatigue. If you are fearful and nervous around needles but would like to experience benefits similar to those of acupuncture, you may want to explore acupressure.

Healing Touch is based on the belief that humans are composed of energy fields that are in constant interaction with the self, environment, and others. The emphasis is on maintaining a balanced flow of energies for good physical, mental, and emotional health. Developed by a nurse named Janet Mentgen in 1980, Healing Touch uses gentle hand techniques to help arrange the energy field and accelerate healing of the body, mind, and spirit. This may sound like simply getting a massage, but it's much more than that. Healing Touch is commonly used to alleviate chronic back pain. The practitioner may focus on the root chakras (spiritual energy centers within the body) to perform hands-on therapeutic skills in opening blocked energies within the back. The practitioner transfers their life-force energy into the client to encourage the healing process to release blocked energy. Healing Touch practitioners may or may not literally touch their patients; they simply use their hands to clear and balance the body's energy field.

It is important to remember that the intention is not to cure anything but rather to create an optimal physical, spiritual, and mental environment so that the body can effectively heal itself. Healing Touch is a complementary therapy, designed to enhance traditional treatments. It has been widely used in nursing homes, hospice facilities, and hospitals to treat pain, cancer symptoms, cardiovascular disease, and stress and to aid in postsurgical recovery.

Healing Touch can also complement other mind-body therapy techniques such as acupressure and massage.

In 1993, Healing Touch was certified by the American Holistic Nurses Association. Today, it's practiced globally in hospitals, nursing schools, clinics, and long-term care centers as a noninvasive approach to healing.

So, what does a typical Healing Touch session look like? A person will sit or lie comfortably while the practitioner becomes calm and focused. The practitioner then sweeps their hands over the person in treatment to scan the person's energy field and detect any imbalances. Next, the practitioner uses gentle touch or off-body touch (near the body but with no direct contact) on various areas of the body to clear the energy. Finally, they will "ground" the patient, bringing them back to an alert state.

Massage therapy focuses on fostering a positive mind-body connection by stimulating sensations arising from the skin. According to *The Oxytocin Factor*, written by Dr. Kerstin Uvnäs-Moberg, massage can release oxytocin—known as the "love hormone." It is released by the hypothalamus and has an important role in reproduction and in triggering labor and the release of breastmilk in mothers. Oxytocin also acts like a neurotransmitter, similar to endorphins, which can lower stress and relieve anxiety.

Massages can also decrease the level of cortisol—a hormone that can cause a number of problems such as depression and high blood pressure if it gets too high for too long. Regular massages can relax tense muscles, release toxins, and reduce physical and emotional stress. Therapeutic application of touch can be a supportive, relaxing treatment that encourages the mind to slow down, while at the same time increasing the body's overall energy and potentially lifting one's spirits. Results can also include improved quality of sleep, concentration, and circulation.

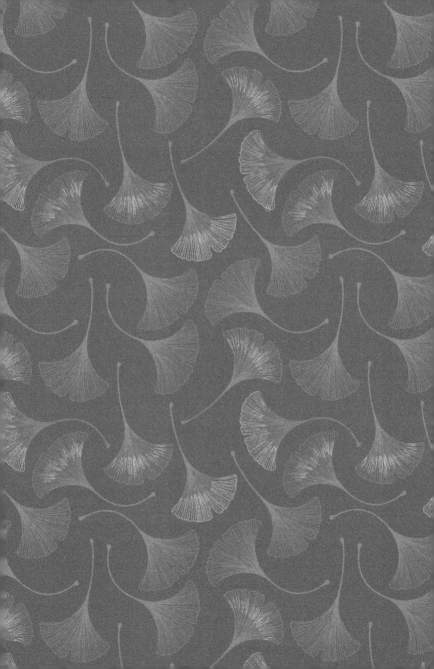

CHAPTER 4

Mind-Body Interventions

The National Center for Complementary and Integrative Health identifies mind-body medicine as a subcategory of complementary and alternative medicine. Mind-body medicine follows a holistic approach that explores the interconnection between the mind and body. (For these interventions, the word "mind" refers to mental states such as thoughts, emotions, attitudes, beliefs, and images in the brain.)

Mind-body interventions include meditation, hypnosis, visualization, guided imagery, and self-hypnosis. These practices are designed to enhance the mind's positive impact on the body with the goal of improving mental, physical, and spiritual health.

According to Dr. Herbert Benson of the Mind/Body Medical Institute of Harvard University, many of the techniques make use of what he calls the "relaxation response." In his book *The Relaxation Response*, Benson describes this as a state in which the body's heart rate, blood pressure, and breathing slow down, facilitating more circulation of oxygen. The body then feels rested, similar to a sleep cycle, for a brief period of time. The relaxation response can help patients with diabetes by lowering the stress response, which in turn lowers a hormone called cortisol. As a result, glucose levels are stabilized and the heart and immune system are protected.

Mind-body interventions can help prevent and relieve stress, which, in turn, helps relieve neck and back pain and nerve conditions such as carpal tunnel syndrome, headaches, and fibromyalgia.

Origins, Growth, and How They're Used Today

Many of these mind-body interventions originate from Eastern healing practices. It is believed that meditation may have first developed in India around 1500 BCE. Meditation was also taught by the Buddha in Southeast Asia over 2,000 years ago. Guided imagery is believed to have been used since the ancient Greeks and Romans.

Mind-body interventions have not always been accepted by conventional Western doctors, who tend to consider the scientific model of medicine to be superior. But during the 20th century, researchers began to study the complex mind-body connection. A study from the *American Journal of Psychiatry* in 2018 shows the connection between being mindful and pain control. For patients who experience chronic pain, it helps to practice mindfulness, which the study describes as being "more in touch with the fullness of one's being through systematic process of self-observation, self-inquiry, and mindful action."

Hans Selye, a researcher who wrote about the subject of mindfulness, published a book in 1956 called *The Stress of Life*. Among other things, he found that when the body is under psychological stress, it responds with a series of physiological and biological changes. Interestingly, he identified stress with the swelling of the frontal cortex, atrophy of the thymus, and gastric ulcers. According to Selye, we have a natural protective response that guides our bodies through acute stress. This is part of our natural survival mechanism. But when this mechanism is constantly caused by the ongoing stress of daily life, it becomes a destructive pattern. The chronic activation of this stress response damages the coping mechanism and can cause premature damage to our bodily functions. In other words, stress in itself is not harmful, and a certain amount is necessary. The problem occurs when we are chronically stressed.

In his book *Integrative Mental Health Care*, Dr. James Lake writes, "Healthy lifestyle choices that are beneficial for mental health also include regular exercise, getting enough sleep, and using relaxation and mindfulness techniques for stress management. In addition to positive lifestyle choices, natural supplements have general beneficial effects on mental health." Chronic stress and post-traumatic stress, anxiety, mood disorders, addiction, and many other ailments plague many people, and conventional medicine is not always successful at treating them. For this reason, mind-body interventions are necessary for helping people manage their stress. In addition, some mind-body interventions have been found to be effective in reducing chronic pain, anxiety, and insomnia. Western science has also found some mind-body interventions to be helpful as complementary practices in the treatment of illness and chronic disease.

The Mind-Body-Spirit Connection

The connection between the mind and the body is both fascinating and worth looking into. Can positive thinking, yoga, or meditation really heal your body as well as your mind? Research studies are showing that mind-body therapies are safe and effective ways of mitigating physical and emotional symptoms. In addition, these practices are safe and noninvasive, which makes them an ideal choice of therapy for patients to integrate in their own self-care. In a 2009 article in the *Journal of Nurse Practitioners*, Mary Koithan shows that patients who participate in these techniques experience certain benefits like the ability to adapt to stress, increased hope, and a more positive outlook on life.

For example, an article from the *International Journal of Yoga* shows that yoga, a system of physical postures, breathing techniques, and sometimes meditation, has been shown to reduce stress and improve the immune system. This thousand-year-old tool is an excellent example of the mind-body connection. Research has also shown that Hatha yoga can help reduce blood sugar levels.

There is a growing body of evidence that shows that people who are stressed are more prone to disease and illness and tend to heal slower than those who are able to maintain their stress levels. Mind-body techniques can play a role in your overall well-being by helping you manage your stress, improve your coping and relaxation skills, and reduce chronic pain. A study published in the *Journal of the American Board of Family Practices* found that several mind-body techniques have been effective in the treatment of coronary artery disease, headaches, chronic back pain, incontinence, hypertension, arthritis, and insomnia. One-third of Americans are living with extreme stress, which is linked to six leading causes of death: cancer, heart disease, lung ailments, accidents, cirrhosis of the liver, and suicide. Mind-body techniques offer an array of strategies that support the body's natural ability to heal itself and decrease stress.

Meditation, Visualization, and Guided Imagery

Meditation is not just a relaxation technique—it's also a strategy for maintaining health, increasing concentration, and training the mind to observe certain thoughts. Amazingly, your brain is able to rewire itself toward happiness, peace, and success. And meditation can help by training your mind to place attention where you want it to go.

For example, a study on brain circuitry conducted by Dr. Richard Davidson of the University of Wisconsin, found that the brain can rewire itself and alter its set points. Dr. Davidson says, "People are not just stuck at their respective set points. We can take advantage of our brain's plasticity and train it to enhance these qualities." He refers to these set points as the original emotions that participants started with. Davidson studied a group of monks who meditated regularly and compared them to a group of people who did not. His amazing finding was that the region of the brain associated with happiness and positivity (the left prefrontal cortex) was more active in the monks.

This is quite a discovery and shows a strong correlation between meditation and quality of life! As with the monks, meditation can help you feel more serene, calm, and at peace. But don't worry. Meditation does not mean you have to sit there like a monk for days on end. That's a common misconception, and meditation definitely isn't just for monks!

Visualization is a technique that requires you to imagine yourself as the main character in a movie you are creating in your mind. This skill is used to stimulate emotions and provide a direct communication with the unconscious part of the mind. Visualization is one of the best ways to get your mind back on track when you feel out of balance. It can have a positive effect on heart rate, blood pressure, and other symptoms caused by stress. It can be used to promote relaxation (which helps lower stress), manage pain, and promote healing.

Guided imagery is similar to visualization in that you use your imagination to create the state you want to be in. The difference is that someone is guiding you. Guided imagery uses words and images to help move your mind and attention away from any current negative feelings such as stress, worry, or pain. It uses all of your senses—touch, hearing, sight, smell, and taste. As with visualization, guided imagery can be used to promote relaxation, manage pain, and promote healing. It can also have a positive effect on heart rate, blood pressure, and other symptoms caused by stress.

Guided imagery has been used by many people to achieve their personal goals. Even elite athletes commonly use this practice to help themselves perform their best. The next time you are feeling stressed or nervous, give this simple and effective technique a try.

You can practice visualization with a therapist or at home with a recorded file or app. An important benefit to this practice is the realization that people can play an active role in their own healing. They feel more empowered knowing that they can find strength in their own minds. This can make a difference in their spirit as well! Both visualization and guided imagery use the power of your imagination to help you relax or relieve symptoms.

Self-Hypnosis

Self-hypnosis is a method you can use to put yourself in a state of deep relaxation, calmness, and heightened awareness. Hypnosis is very similar to the mental states you can achieve during meditation and yoga, and it can be very pleasant. Your mind and body are relaxed, but at the same time, you are extremely alert, focused, and in touch with reality. These are the main features that distinguish it from daydreaming, meditation, sleep, or visualization. Hypnosis can also help you minimize old limiting beliefs and behavior patterns that are no longer serving you. The goal is to help make room for new positive beliefs. This is why it's commonly used along with alternative healing therapies to release past traumas, enhance memory, release fear, and even improve self-esteem. In other words, hypnosis can help uncover and bring into light the stored information or experiences from the subconscious mind.

Hypnosis can be guided by a professionally trained hypnotherapist, but self-hypnosis, as the term implies, is conducted by you. There are many resources available to guide you in this process, including online videos, audios, and books (see Resources on page 199). Note that during a session of self-hypnosis you can bring yourself out of the hypnotic state if there are any interruptions that require your immediate attention. You are in complete control.

The American Medical Association, the American Dental Association, and the American Psychological Association have all recognized hypnotherapy as a valid therapeutic modality. Hypnosis can help with many issues such as back pain, weight loss, addictions, and unhealthy habits such as smoking. Hypnosis can also be highly beneficial to relieve stress or to clear your mind before an important work presentation. The key is to calm the mind down, which is commonly achieved when combined with positive affirmations.

A Note of Caution

Self-hypnosis may not be suitable if you are experiencing mental illness or taking medications for anxiety. Consult with your physician before trying self-hypnosis. If you have any questions or concerns, you might want to attend a few sessions with a qualified hypnotist to go over the technique before trying it on your own.

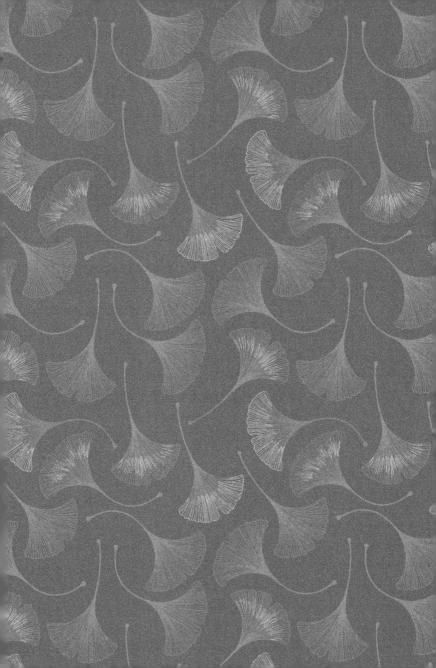

CHAPTER 5

Biologically Based Therapies

The National Center for Complementary and Integrative Health (NCCIH) defines biologically based therapies as alternative treatments that use substances found in nature such as herbs, foods, and vitamins. These therapies include a wide range of treatments, from aromatherapy to herbal medicine, and make use of many different natural substances including dietary supplements, herbs, vitamins, and probiotics. There are healing powers in herbs, foods, and vitamins; they can have a profound effect on the way we feel both mentally and physically. In this chapter, we will concentrate on aromatherapy, flower essences, essential oils, and herbs.

Origins, Growth, and How They're Used Today

The history of herbal medicine probably started in India over 4,000 years ago and then spread to China. Traditional Chinese Medicine developed a strong philosophical viewpoint on health, with common treatments including herbal medicine. Knowledge of herbal medicine also traveled to the Middle East and eventually across the globe. According to the NCCIH, the interest in and use of natural products in the United States have grown considerably in the last couple of decades. A comprehensive National Health Interview Survey found that the complementary health products most commonly used by American adults and children were fish oil and omega-3 supplements.

Today, some conventional doctors are more open to recommending medicinal herbs, given reasonable evidence of safety and effectiveness. Some doctors are even recommending these herbs in addition to prescribing drugs. Herbs are often used to treat a variety of ailments including stress, infertility, and hormonal imbalance. While herbal medicine can be very beneficial, it is considered most effective when used in conjunction with other natural treatments such as nutritional modification, movement, and stress reduction. Aromatherapy and flower essences also have a variety of uses in holistic medicine including massage therapy, topical applications, and inhalation.

It's important to note that the market for herbs and dietary supplements is not regulated as strictly as pharmaceuticals. In addition, there are many unsubstantiated claims made for herbal remedies. For these two reasons, it's best if you purchase from reputable brands. Look for herbal preparations that have been wild-crafted, which ensures the herbs are ethically harvested and cultivated organically. Dietary supplements are often "prescribed" by naturopaths and nutritionists. They typically contain dietary ingredients including vitamins, minerals, herbs, amino acids, probiotics, or other botanical constituents.

The Mind-Body-Spirit Connection

Mother Nature has given us precious gifts in the form of herbs, food, and vitamins. Biologically based therapies can help you restore balance of the mind, body, and spirit.

There are thousands of different species of plants and foods available in nature. They offer nourishment to your body, food for your soul, communication for your brain, and restoration of your overall health. Foods such as turmeric and ginger can relieve inflammation and help your joints feel better. Foods such as pomegranates and beets can improve blood flow and can be beneficial for people who wish to alleviate back pain or leg pain.

In his book *Foods that Fight Pain,* Dr. Neal Barnard reports that specific compounds in some foods, including fruits like cherries and spices like turmeric, can fight common pains such as migraines, arthritis, and menstrual cramps. These types of pain are caused by inflammation brought on by hormones that are released into the body. According to Dr. Barnard, these foods appear to have a positive influence over these hormones.

In part 3 of this book, you will find some food remedies to help with digestive-related conditions such as irritable bowel syndrome. For instance, probiotics (live microorganisms that are good for your gut) are found in fermented foods such as sauerkraut, yogurt, and kefir. These bacteria can help improve physical functions, such as increasing your body's ability to absorb iron. Interestingly, probiotics can also have a positive effect on cognition, emotion, and behavior. Studies have shown that certain strains can help reduce stress by reducing levels of the hormone cortisol.

Plants (and the herbs and spices that come from them) have many healing powers. Turmeric, one of the most well-researched herbal medicines in the world, is a great example. It can be eaten or taken as a supplement and has many benefits, such as reducing inflammation and preventing heart disease. Ginger is another good example of an herb with healing powers. It has been used for centuries by Ayurveda practitioners to treat neurological conditions such as nausea and headaches.

Vitamins and minerals are nutrients found in food, and we need them to stay healthy and vibrant. When they are missing from your diet, you can replace them with supplements. Vitamins and minerals attempt to supply the body with the proper nutrients that are critical for organ function. Certain vitamins may facilitate healing when the immune system is weakened by infection. Similarly, they can be used postsurgically to accelerate healing and prevent the chance of getting infections.

Today, many practitioners are recommending positive changes in nutritional self-care based on advances in nutritional science and emerging nutritional systems of healing.

Aromatherapy, Essential Oils, and Flower Essences

Aromatherapy is a holistic treatment that uses natural plant extracts, called essential oils, to promote healing and well-being.

Essential oils are concentrated plant extracts that retain the natural smell and flavor—the essence—of their source.

Have you ever noticed as you peel an orange that there are tiny amounts of oil residue on your fingers? If you put your finger to your nose and inhale the citrus smell, does it feel invigorating? That is an example of what essential oils can do. Smell is one of the most forceful, evocative senses. Aromatherapy builds on the power of smell, using essential oils for wellness and healing. Aromatherapy isn't just about smelling essential oils, though. There are many different ways to apply these oils including diffusers, balms applied directly to the skin, steams, and inhalers.

Essential oils have a long history of use to support common ailments. Their wide range of uses includes treating skincare issues, preventing cold and flu symptoms, improving mood, and alleviating symptoms of respiratory conditions. For example, eucalyptus essential oils have a decongestant property that simulates oxygen uptake in the cells, making it one of the most powerful respiratory supporters.

Since essential oils are highly aromatic, many of their benefits are obtained through inhalation. The vapors stimulate your olfactory nerves, which send signals to the limbic system (the part of the brain that controls emotions), amygdala, and hippocampus (the control center in the brain for memory and emotions).

Flower essences are created by soaking flowers in water to "imprint" their energy. This energy is preserved in alcohol or vegetable glycerin. To understand how flower essence can heal the body, you must first understand the theory of flower remedies developed by Edward Bach, an English doctor, bacteriologist, homeopath, and spiritual writer in the 1930s. Bach believed that our bodies are fields of vibrating energy and that flowers have their own vibrations that can be therapeutic. You can transfer these vibrations to your body by placing flower essence on your tongue or applying it to your body.

Bach also believed that we are born as perfect human beings. As we grow older, the stress of daily life causes an accumulation of unhealthy patterns as we try to cope with the stress. This eventually causes a spiritual imbalance and misalignment, which then manifests as disease. Muscles can tighten up, causing tension. And wherever there is tension, there's a blockage of flow in energy. Flower essences fill our energy field with vibrations that can help loosen the energy blocks that prevent us from vibrating at our highest frequency of pure health. Flower essences can address underlying emotions by releasing unwanted patterns that don't serve you and attracting the things that do serve you. Flower essences can act as a catalyst for positive changes at an emotional level, such as feeling more joy, creativity, and connection on a spiritual level.

Herbal Remedies

Herbal remedies are plants and herbs that are used to help prevent or cure disease. Herbal medicine, which features the use of herbal remedies, is the most widely practiced form of medicine in the world. We have been incorporating herbs into our medical treatment for centuries to support vitality and connect us with Mother Nature. Today, many practitioners from holistic nutritionists to naturopathic doctors and herbalists are incorporating herbal remedies as a way to help their patients support whole-body wellness.

Here are a few examples of herbal remedies and their wellness-supporting properties:

Elderberry supports the immune system and can reduce the duration of a cold or flu.

Ginger root has been found to support immune function and cardiovascular health. It is also well known for its beneficial digestive properties.

Chamomile is one of the most widely used herbal remedies and is used for many common ailments. It contains antioxidants and has anti-inflammatory properties. Many people also drink chamomile tea before bed to help them sleep.

St. John's wort contains two active compounds called hypericin and hyperforin that are known to have calming effects. This herb is used as an antidepressant since it has a calming effect and can reduce anxiety. Hyperforin can also decrease inflammation and has antibacterial properties.

Ashwagandha is an herb that may help the body adapt to stress and aging. It can also help people stay focused, sleep better, and reduce feelings of anxiety or depression.

 Triphala has been part of traditional Ayurvedic medicine since ancient times. It is used as a digestive tonic and for detoxification.

 Sage has played a significant role in the healing and spiritual ceremonies of indigenous cultures for thousands of years. An important tool to connect the physical and spiritual world, it also smells wonderful and has a calming effect.

Herbal supplements come in different forms and can be found dried, chopped, as a liquid, or in a capsule. You can even grow many of them in your backyard! Using herbs and spices that have disease-preventive effects in foods is one of the best ways to take advantage of their healing power. By having a well-stocked holistic medicine cabinet that includes a few herbal staples, you will be on your way to supporting your body's stress response, immune system, mood, and wellness through the holistic power of healing plants and herbs.

Must-Have Items

Here are some staples you should stock up on so you can take full advantage of the holistic healing remedies in this book:

ESSENTIAL OILS

Clary sage	Lavender	Vetiver
Clove	Lemon	Ylang-ylang
Eucalyptus	Peppermint	
Frankincense	Tea tree oil	

FLOWER ESSENCES

Cherry plum	Larch	Star of Bethlehem
Clematis	Olive	White chestnut
Holly	Rock rose	Wild oat
Impatiens		

HERBS

Aloe vera	Lavender	Rosemary
Chamomile	Nettle	St. John's wort
Elderberry	Peppermint	Turmeric
Ginger		

Nutrition Therapy

Nutrition therapy is a healing practice based on the belief that whole foods—foods that have not been processed and are in their natural state—provide us with the essential substances needed to keep the body in a vibrant state of health. This practice complements holistic health by focusing on the whole body, including the digestive, immune, endocrine, and cardiovascular systems.

Nutrition therapy programs all agree on one basic recommendation: Eat nutrient-dense whole foods, including raw fruits and vegetables, beans, legumes, nuts, seeds, whole grains, pastured organic animal products, and wild fish. Nutrients can be found in animal and plant sources and are broken down into macronutrients (protein, fats, carbohydrates) and micronutrients (vitamins, minerals, antioxidants, phytochemicals). Nutritional therapy teaches that food should be consumed in its whole, unaltered form. When you eat foods that are still in their most natural form, you reap the full benefits of critical enzymes and phytochemicals (chemicals found in plant foods that may prevent cancer and heart disease), boost your immune system, and slow down the aging process. For instance, raw vegetables provide more nutrients than their cooked versions.

One of the most important phytochemicals are antioxidants, which help fight disease. Some examples of antioxidants are vitamin C, which is found in oranges, and beta-carotene, which is found in carrots. A growing body of clinical evidence suggests that consumption of phytochemicals from plant-based foods such as fruits, vegetables, grain, and tea is linked to protection from chronic disease including cancer and heart disease.

According to Dr. Joel Fuhrman, who researches and specializes in preventing and reversing disease through nutritional and natural methods, a diet based on the principles of nutrition therapy can actually prevent and reverse chronic conditions like diabetes. In one study published in the *American Journal of Lifestyle Medicine*, Fuhrman found that participants who adhered to his dietary guidelines over an average span of three years experienced weight loss and lowering of cholesterol (both risk factors of cardiovascular disease).

CHAPTER 6

Manipulative and Body-Based Therapies

Manipulative and body-based therapies comprise a system of treatment that uses manual manipulation or movement of certain body parts to fix or improve structural imbalances of the joints, bones, and soft tissues.

This type of therapy focuses on the overall structure and systems of the human body, with an emphasis on the soft tissue, bones and joints, lymphatic system, and circulatory system.

Practices include acupuncture, osteopathic manipulation, chiropractic adjustments, body movement, reflexology, and massage (covered in chapter 3).

Origins, Growth, and How They're Used Today

Acupuncture originated in China roughly 2,500 years ago, and it's one of the oldest manipulative and body-based therapies still used today. It involves inserting thin needles through a person's skin at various acupressure points on the body, with the goal of reaching a harmonious balance of yin and yang to allow the life force known as qi to flow throughout the body.

Acupuncture has been continually used in Asia since ancient times, but it didn't become well known in the United States until about 1950 when the US Food and Drug Administration (FDA) classified acupuncture needles as medical instruments. According to 2007 National Health Interview Survey data, its popularity has continued to grow since then with an estimated 6.5 percent of Americans using it to relieve pain, headaches, arthritis, and fibromyalgia. Chiropractic adjustments and osteopathic manipulation were developed in the early 1900s, and both require extensive formal training in the anatomy and physiology of the human body. Both practices believe that the human body is self-regulating, meaning it has the ability to heal itself.

While chiropractic therapists only adjust the spine, osteopaths focus on all joints. Osteopathic manipulation was developed by a physician named Andrew Taylor Still, who was frustrated with the toxic side effects of medications used for spinal meningitis in the 1800s. He founded the American School of Osteopathy, where he taught and promoted healing by manipulating bones to allow free circulation of blood and balanced nerve functioning.

Chiropractic medicine was founded in 1896 by Daniel David Palmer, who discovered the principle of chiropractic when he helped a janitor hear again by manipulating his neck. Palmer established the Palmer School of Cure, now known as the Palmer College of Chiropractic in Davenport, Iowa.

Osteopathic adjustments have provided aid for people with spinal and joint conditions, lower back pain, arthritis, allergies, chronic fatigue syndrome, headaches, sciatica, and inflammation of the nerves. Chiropractic adjustments can help with back pain, neck pain, headaches, mobility, flexibility, and subluxation (a condition in which the spine is in misalignment). Today, there are more than 70,000 active chiropractic licenses in the United States and over 7,000 in Canada. According to a report based on the 2017 National Health Interview Survey (NHIS), the use of chiropractors increased from 9.1% in 2012 to 10.3% in 2017 for adults in the United States. Spinal manipulation therapy is currently used by osteopathic surgeons, chiropractors, and physical therapists with the goal of relieving pain and improving physical functioning. It is used to treat conditions including sciatica, lower back pain, neck pain, and headaches.

Tai chi and qigong are ancient Chinese movement practices that use postures and gentle rhythmic movement as well as mental focus, breathing, and relaxation. Originating roughly 3,000 years ago, they have been practiced continually in Asia since then. Tai chi, a form of martial arts that emphasizes gentleness, was widely used in China to improve balance, immunity, and reduce stress. Based on a 2002 national survey on Americans' use of complementary and alternative medicine, about 2.5 million people use tai chi and half a million people use qigong for health reasons.

Yoga, another ancient movement practice, originated in India about 5,000 years ago and has been practiced there continually since then. It came to the West in 1893 but didn't gain popularity until 1950 when yoga teacher Richard Hittleman emphasized the physical benefits of yoga to Americans.

Originally called zone therapy, reflexology was created in 1913 by Dr. William Fitzgerald. In the 1930s the methodology was revised by Eunice Ingham, who renamed it reflexology. The therapy is based on the idea that every organ in the body is connected to a certain area on the foot and that placing pressure on these areas can help heal whichever organ is in pain. Essential oils are commonly used. Reflexology is now used in spas and is also being taught in universities across the United States. As reflexology gained greater acceptance as a credible complementary therapy, the American Reflexology Certification Board, an independent testing agency for the field of reflexology, was created to help maintain high standards of care. Today, reflexology is used to complement other treatments for anxiety, asthma, cancer, headaches, and diabetes. Overall, manipulative and body-based therapies are used today to treat a variety of conditions including arthritis and joint pain, headaches, neck and shoulder pain, lower back pain, accident-related and sports injuries, stress, fibromyalgia, and even anxiety.

The Mind-Body-Spirit Connection

Manipulative and body-based therapies can help you connect with your body by restoring you to optimal health and wellness in a noninvasive way. These practices involve moving the body in a way that allows you to understand that physically restrictive patterns can be changed and improved.

Chiropractic manipulation focuses on the relationship between the spine and its function and how it affects the rest of the body. Chiropractors perform adjustments on the spine or other parts of the body to correct alignment problems, alleviate pain, improve functions like walking, and support the body's natural ability to heal itself.

Tai chi may help improve balance and stability and reduce back pain and knee pain. Conditions that could benefit from this modality of healing include fibromyalgia, Parkinson's disease, and osteoporosis. A 2018 randomized controlled trial, supported by the National Center for Complementary and Integrative Health, on 226 adults with fibromyalgia showed that frequent practice of tai chi reduced symptom severity more than aerobic exercise. Because the movements are slow, tai chi is considered safe and unlikely to cause injury. It can be done in a group setting or at home by watching an online video.

Yoga is another meditative movement practice that can benefit both the mind and body. There are various types of yoga exercises, and they all share similar elements that combine physical postures, breathing techniques, and relaxation. Vinyasa yoga is a popular type of practice that helps improve muscle tone, strength, and flexibility. You're more likely to see this type of yoga being shared on social media. It's a dynamic practice that can also boost one's confidence and self-image. Hatha yoga typically involves a set of physical postures and breathing techniques and is practiced at a slower pace than Vinyasa. These postures (or yoga poses) are designed to align the muscles and bones and, most important, open energy channels so that energy can flow freely throughout the body.

Both styles of body movement teach breathing techniques that allow you to be more present, be aware of your surroundings, and control your thoughts. Mastering these techniques can help you feel more calm and centered, lower your stress levels, and generally live a more peaceful life.

Movement and Exercise

Movement and exercise can be an important component of holistic healing. Exercise can keep your body fit while contributing to a sense of balance and leave you feeling relaxed and invigorated afterward. Yoga is an amazing exercise that rewards the body with a good workout while promoting balanced health and a calm mind. Tai chi is a form of martial arts that emphasizes deep breathing, deliberate slow movements, and physical balance, and it can help reduce stress. There is also qigong, which is a blend of martial arts and yoga. Qigong is a type of exercise system used particularly for mental and physical training. It emphasizes flexibility, gentle movements, mindfulness, and meditative breathing.

Incorporating exercise into your daily routine can help reduce the risk of chronic illness. For example, exercise helps improve insulin sensitivity, which is great for the treatment and prevention of diabetes. Also, it effectively reduces inflammation, which has been shown to be the root cause of many health issues. Daily movement can be an amazing antiaging tool as well. Simple exercises, like hiking, are an excellent way to maintain a healthy body weight and improve balance, bone mineral mass, and overall flexibility. Bone loss is a natural occurrence as we age, but exercising can help build strong bones and decelerate bone loss. Strategic and deliberate types of movement including tai chi and yoga can help with balance and flexibility, which can reduce your risk of falling or getting injured.

Exercising can also enhance your mental health and even relieve symptoms of depression. When your body is engaged in movement, the brain releases endorphins, dopamine, and serotonin, known as the "feel good" or "happiness" hormones. Raising the levels of these brain chemicals can boost your mood and improve sleep and overall health. Endorphins help you deal with stress and reduce feelings of pain. They're made by the central nervous system and act on the opiate receptors in the brain, which boost feelings of pleasure and decrease pain.

There is a lot of flexibility in choosing the right exercise program. Movement can be as simple and short or as long and intense as you choose. Rebounding, for example, is a fun and low-impact practice that helps drain the lymphatic system—all you have to do is jump on a trampoline for 20 minutes! There are many other fun, low-impact movements such as dancing, walking your dog, gardening, hiking, and swimming. As long as you are committed to daily movement, you will experience a positive impact on your mind, body, and spirit.

CHAPTER 7

Energy Therapies

Energy therapies are a variety of techniques meant to heal a person by using their body's life-force energy. The goal of energy therapy is to improve the flow and balance of energy fields in and around the body, resulting in health and well-being, reduced pain symptoms, quicker healing, and improvement in other related symptoms.

There are many types of and applications for energy therapy. In this chapter, we will focus on a few of the most effective practices that can be easily incorporated into your alternative healing plan. With this information, you can make an informed and motivated decision to try them out!

Maybe you were involved in a car accident. Or you've been emotionally hurt by a family member or close friend. Perhaps you are grieving. When you are physically injured or have suffered emotional pain, there may be a stagnation of energy in your body. In other words, the flow of energy is being blocked, which can lead to illness. Energy therapy uses different forms of energy to heal, including electromagnetic and subtle energy.

Origins, Growth, and How They're Used Today

The origins of energy therapy go back to the 1920s when Japanese Zen Buddhist Dr. Mikao Usui rediscovered the ancient healing practice known today as Reiki. In 1936, an American named Hawayo Takata trained in Reiki and became a Reiki master. She later introduced Reiki to the United States.

The word Reiki comes from the Japanese words *rei* (universal) and *ki* (life energy). In this practice, a Reiki master or other practitioner transfers energy to a patient by placing their hands on or near the areas of the patient's body in need of an energy boost. They also use crystals and chakra healing wands to enable healing. Although initially there was some controversy around energy healing since it is difficult to prove its effectiveness through scientific studies, the practice has continued to gain popularity in recent years. A survey conducted in 2007 reported that in the previous year, 1.2 million adults and 161,000 children in the United States received one or more energy healing sessions such as Reiki.

Reiki is also gaining wider acceptance in the conventional medical establishment and is currently used in hospitals, hospices, private wellness centers, and at home. Because of the positive results that have been demonstrated and due to patient requests, Reiki has gained credibility and is being used as a complementary treatment for anxiety, chronic pain, and cancer.

Reiki can also be done at home as a form of self-healing or through distant healing (where the healer and patient are in different locations). Reiki is similar to Healing Touch (covered in chapter 3) and requires an attunement, or a connection or initiation between the Reiki student and the natural universal energy, before a practitioner can practice on a patient. According to the International Center for Reiki Training, attunement is a connection that allows Reiki to flow through the student's body for self-treatments or treatment of others. According to experts in energy healing, when your aura (the magnetic field that surrounds each human being) is blocked, problems can develop, including mood disorders like depression and anxiety. Your physical health can be affected, too. These imbalances can leave you feeling exhausted, disconnected, negative, and "off."

Today, many people work with Reiki practitioners to cleanse their auras. But this can also be done at home, using a variety of practices such as smudging, a technique that requires the burning of a small bundle of dried sage. According to Reiki teachings, smudging removes unwanted and negative energy in the house and around your physical body.

Crystals may look pretty but they are also functional and useful in energy healing. In Chinese feng shui, the natural spiritual energies of crystals are used to amplify and balance the flow of qi throughout your home. Each crystal has different structures and properties to promote health and well-being. Crystals and gems can also be used by Reiki masters for their healing qualities, beauty, and ability to conduct energy. For centuries, people have placed crystals on the body's chakras (also known as energy centers) to release energy blockages. For example, amethyst is used to treat headaches. Tiger's eye is most common for relieving stress; its earthy features make the crystal very grounding. Some people carry the crystals around to aid in their own healing or give them to others who need energy healing.

Science has proven that our bodies actually project their own magnetic fields and that our cells communicate through electromagnetic frequencies. The use of magnetic fields originated around 4000 BCE when Hindus treated disease with naturally magnetized stones called lodestones. In 2000 BCE, Chinese doctors used these lodestones on acupuncture points. In ancient Greece, Hippocrates reportedly used magnets to alleviate patients' pain.

In the 1980s, the first FDA-approved pulsed electromagnetic field (PEMF) system was introduced to treat bone fractures. Dr. William Pawluk, a family physician and holistic health practitioner, studied PEMFs extensively and found that PEMF treatments can give the cells in our bodies a tune-up that can help with cell dysfunction. A study also shows how PEMF treatments can stimulate blood flow to improve circulation due to movement of ions. According to Pawluk, increased circulation is one of the primary benefits of PEMF therapy in helping the body heal, increasing nutrients, and improving immune functions. This method has grown in popularity as people are seeking alternatives for healing. Some hospitals in the United States and Europe now offer these healing methods in addition to their standard medical care.

The Mind-Body-Spirit Connection

To truly understand the powerful benefits of energy healing, it's important to understand the concept of subtle energy, which is described in Donna Eden's book *Energy Medicine* as "electro-magnetic wavelengths, rates of vibration, and patterns of pulsation—the dynamic infrastructure of the body." By examining subtle energy, you will see that many physical discomforts experienced in the body are caused by some form of blockage. You can then take the appropriate course of action, either a home remedy or a session with an energy healer, to alleviate the discomfort you are experiencing.

According to experts in energy healing, pain is a common manifestation of a blockage of subtle energy. It's harder to pinpoint than the kind of physiological pain that we experience, for example, from accidentally touching a hot stove. For instance, have you ever felt a deep, mysterious pain inside your body? You try to describe it to your doctor, and after a few ultrasound and MRI tests, you are left with no diagnosis. It is possible you are dealing with a blockage of subtle energy.

Tension is another common blockage of subtle energy. If you have tight muscles, a massage can help release that energy through the muscles, internal organs, or tissues. This can cause a temporary release of tension in the body. Notice sometimes that your body feels stiff when you try to move the next day following a massage session; that's the natural process of releasing blocked energy.

Many factors can contribute to blockages of our energy flow including nutrition, environmental pollution, lifestyle, stress, fear, negative emotions, negative experiences, and childhood trauma. By removing these blockages in the energy field and rebalancing the energy, the body can return to its level of balance. Energy healing can transform your life and benefit you physically, emotionally, and spiritually.

Energy Healing and Reiki

Energy healing is a traditional healing system that aims to restore the balance and flow of energy throughout the body, mind, and soul. **Reiki** is a subtle and effective form of energy healing using spiritually guided life-force energy.

According to Reiki masters, energy is meant to flow wherever it is most needed. A practitioner passes energy from the universal energy source to the client. He or she can remove negative energies as well. Some patients report sensations of cold, warmth, tingling, rejuvenation, and a decrease in symptoms. People who receive Reiki typically describe it as intensively relaxing.

The National Center for Complementary and Integrative Health has suggested that Reiki can be used alongside other treatments, particularly for those with more serious health issues. This powerful flow of energy can offer immediate relief, releasing tension and stress. It helps shift the body from a stressed fight-or-flight state to a state of relaxation. As we know, less stress in the body will lead to other benefits. Your body's healing mechanisms can receive a boost and function optimally. Other physical responses, such as a decrease in blood pressure and heart rate and an increase in immune function, can occur.

The beautiful thing about Reiki is that after a few sessions with a certified Reiki master, you can incorporate what you've learned and do it yourself. Whenever you're in a situation that requires you to re-center yourself, you can use Reiki to calm yourself. It can really help energize and provide clarity of mind.

PART 3

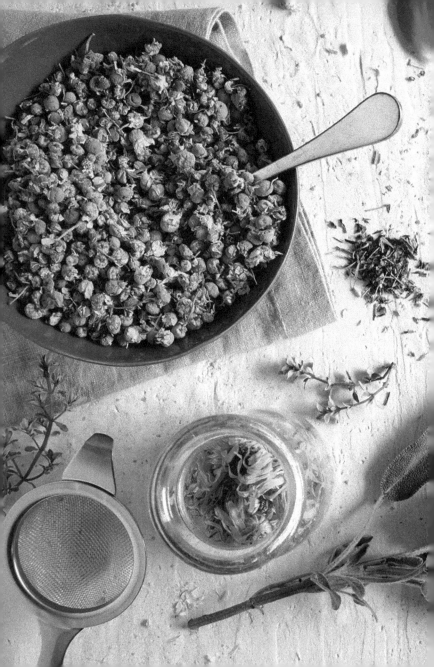

Remedies for Health and Healing

Now we've reached the exciting part—the actual holistic healing remedies!

In this part you'll find a list of 26 common issues, conditions, and ailments, arranged alphabetically for your convenience. Three possible at-home treatments are provided for each issue, including natural remedies and alternative practices. In addition, you'll find a brief description of the issue, condition, or ailment and its symptoms.

Words of Wisdom

Understanding your health and taking responsibility for looking after yourself will ensure that you have the best chance at healing your condition. This involves adopting a holistic strategy that encompasses the whole body, mind, and spirit, rather than just treating symptoms. To truly achieve wellness from a holistic perspective, you have to view and support your body as the incredible machine that it is—one with the powerful ability to heal itself. Your body wants to heal. It wants to get back to balance and harmony—and this should be your goal. As long as you work with the laws of nature, nourish it properly, and provide the right environment, your body can often heal itself naturally. It's also important to connect with the natural world, from which there is so much to learn. Optimal health comes from embracing the healing power of plants as food and medicine and honoring the interconnectivity of all living things.

Healing is different for everybody. There is no single correct approach for every human and, likewise, no cookie-cutter treatment plan for every ailment. Holistic healing is a not a linear process; there will be ups and downs and sometimes more detours. Stay focused and positive, and commit to trying new remedies that will allow you to support your whole being, restore your health, and unleash your body's innate intelligence and ability to heal itself. And remember to enjoy the process!

Holistic Healing Remedies for Common Health Issues, Conditions, and Ailments

In the following section, you'll find a wide range of home remedies, from essential oils used in aromatherapy to meditation practices that can effectively treat common ailments and conditions. Some of these home remedies are drawn from the teaching of the two most ancient holistic healing systems: Traditional Chinese Medicine and Ayurveda. For example, the central message of Ayurveda is "Let food be your medicine and kitchen be your first pharmacy."

In selecting the healing tools and practices in this section, I chose to emphasize herbs, essential oils, plants, and food because they have been used since ancient times. These medicinal ingredients should be available at local health food stores. You probably already have a few of the medicinal herbs in your kitchen. The remedies are also simple to include in your health regimen.

Mother Nature has gifted us with an abundance of useful and special medicinal plants. You must use them with respect. Don't overuse them, and keep in mind that due to bioindividuality, each remedy can have different results with each person. So if one remedy doesn't provide the immediate result that you want, try a different one. Be patient, stay positive, and keep an open mind as you try these remedies out.

This section of the book is intended to be a resource and to offer you information you can use to dig deeper and inspire you on your own road to healing. *But please remember, it should not be taken as medical advice. Use it as a resource and seek advice from your primary doctor before trying any new remedy, especially if you are currently taking any medications.* Some natural products, as amazing as they are, may interact negatively with some prescription drugs.

ACNE/SKIN

Acne is a common skin condition that can occur at any age. According to the American Academy of Dermatology, acne occurs when oil mixes with dead skin and clogs the pores. Your body makes sebum, an oil that keeps your skin from drying out. Typically, skin cells are supposed to shed and get replaced with new cells. Sometimes, sebum can get stuck to the dead cells and cause the pores to clog up. In addition, bacteria can enter the pores and start to proliferate, causing a breakout of pimples. It can make the skin look red due to the inflammation.

In her book *Clean Skin from Within*, Dr. Trevor Cates discusses the underlying issues with particular skin types that are prone to breaking out. According to Dr. Cates, the root causes of acne are blood sugar imbalance, hormonal imbalance, microbiome disturbance, and inflammation. From a holistic perspective, to heal chronic acne, you can focus on eating meals with balanced macronutrients of healthy fats, carbohydrates, and protein. Support your hormones by eating foods high in fiber such as cruciferous vegetables (broccoli and cauliflower) and omega-3s (fish). Lowering your stress is also important in balancing your hormones.

Nutritional Therapy: Rejuvenating Face Mask

Papaya is rich in vitamins A, C, and E that help keep the skin soft. Kiwis also have vitamin C and alpha hydroxy acid (AHA), a natural acid that helps support skin health by exfoliating your skin. Honey has antimicrobial properties and helps balance sebum production. Adding in essential oils like tea tree oil is optional but may help since it has antimicrobial and anti-inflammatory properties.

It's best to put this mask on at night because AHA can cause photosensitivity. This gentle and natural DIY mask can be applied daily or weekly.

- 1 small kiwi (or 1 tablespoon papaya)
- 1 tablespoon plain yogurt
- 1 teaspoon oatmeal flour
- 1 teaspoon raw honey
- 1 drop tea tree essential oil (optional)

1. Peel the kiwi and put it (or the papaya) in a bowl. Use a fork to mash it.

2. Add the yogurt, oatmeal flour, honey, and tea tree oil (if using). Gently mix together.

3. Gently apply the mask evenly onto clean skin. Leave it on for 10 to 20 minutes.

4. Rinse with warm water.

Tip: If you don't have oatmeal flour, simply put oatmeal in a blender or coffee grinder and blend until it has a fine texture, like flour.

Nutritional Therapy: Tropical Piña Colada Smoothie

Papayas and pineapples are amazing fruits for skin health. Both of these tropical fruits contain vitamins C and A, as well as skin-enhancing nutrients like potassium and fiber. Papayas also contain papain, an enzyme that supports your digestive system. Pineapple contains bromelain, an enzyme that helps digest protein, which is helpful in exfoliating dead skin cells. This smoothie is not only refreshing and delicious but provides a balanced amount of carbohydrates, healthy fats, protein, and fiber.

- 1 cup papaya (or a mix of ½ cup papaya and ½ cup pineapple)
- 1 cup spinach
- 1 tablespoon chia seeds or flaxseeds
- 3 to 4 mint leaves
- 1 tablespoon lemon juice (about ½ lemon)
- 2 cups unsweetened coconut milk or hemp milk
- 1 serving collagen powder or plant-based protein powder
- 2 pitted dates or ¼ banana (optional, to sweeten)
- ½-inch piece ginger (optional, to help your body digest the smoothie)

1. Put the papaya, spinach, chia seeds, and mint leaves in a high-speed blender.

Continued >

Nutritional Therapy: Tropical Piña Colada Smoothie continued

2. Add the lemon juice, coconut milk, collagen powder, dates or banana (if using), and ginger (if using).

3. Blend for 30 to 60 seconds until smooth.

4. Pour into a tall glass and enjoy. You can store any left-over smoothie in the refrigerator for up to 2 days.

Exercise Therapy: Rebounding

Daily movement and exercise is essential in helping your skin clear up because it enhances detoxification and increases blood flow and lymph circulation. Exercise is also good for your skin since it helps combat stress and boost your immune system, which can also result in fewer break-outs. Cardiovascular exercise can include running on the pavement or treadmill for 30 minutes. You can also try this rebounding exercise if you have a small trampoline.

1. Stand on the trampoline with your feet spread out about shoulder-width apart.

2. Relax your arms by your sides.

3. Gently bounce up and down for two to five minutes to warm up your body. Your arms should be slightly bent at the elbow. As you bounce, your feet do not have to be very high up. The ideal distance is about 12 inches. Breathe deeply as you bounce.

4. To increase your heart rate, you can do jumping jacks by extending your arms out and bringing them up over your head. You can also raise your knees up toward your chest as you bounce. Do this for five minutes.

5. For advanced movements, you can do alternating high knees. Raise your right knee high and then lower it. Then raise your left knee and lower it. Alternate between the left and right knees as you increase the speed, similar to running. Do this for two-minute intervals.

ADDICTION

Addiction can take many forms, from eating disorders to drug and alcohol abuse. What all addictions have in common is the damage that is done to the body. Holistic treatment for substance addiction (e.g., cocaine and alcohol) focuses on rebuilding the immune system and dealing with and conquering depression.

Conventional addiction treatment programs can include joining a group, seeing a therapist, or taking medication. The downside to breaking an addiction by taking anti-anxiety medications or tranquilizers is that they can have severe side effects down the road or even replace one addiction with another. Withdrawal symptoms and side effects can also cause other health problems.

The good news is that there are many natural ways to help break an addiction. Holistic approaches such as meditation, exercise, and massage therapy can help people during rehabilitation while supporting their psychological and physical health. These treatments can help reduce negative behaviors and address a broad range of factors that play a role in the root of the addiction.

Nature Therapy: Forest Bathing

Grounding is a way to reconnect with nature and can have a powerful impact on symptoms associated with addiction such as depression or tension. Forest bathing, also known as *shinrin-yoku*, is an excellent way to practice grounding. The environment of trees, clear air, and greenery can all promote a lower concentration of the stress hormone cortisol while also lowering blood pressure.

1. Identify your ideal forest bathing location.
2. Leave behind your phone, or turn it off so you will not get distracted.
3. Walk or hike until you reach a spot where you're surrounded by nature and trees.
4. Slow down as you move through the forest.
5. Take long, deep breaths.
6. Stop and stand in any spot. Take in your surroundings using all your senses. What do you smell? How do you feel? Be observant to your surroundings. Pay attention to the colors of nature.

Tip: Try to do this a few times a week to benefit from the calming effect on your cortisol levels, which will certainly enhance your healing journey. To practice grounding, take off your shoes and walk barefoot. Alternatively, you can lie down flat on the ground while doing action #6.

Exercise Therapy: Using Water Barbells

Exercise is one of the most important ways to kick an addiction. It's known as a natural antidepressant for good reason. Exercise prompts your body to release its own psychoactive substances known as endorphins, which trigger the brain's reward pathway. This is an important consideration if you are trying to cope with addiction.

Exercise also provides the brain with support, teaching it to recognize that there are other ways to stimulate the reward center without using substances. Developing an exercise routine can also replace destructive addictive patterns that once consumed your time. For this exercise you'll need a set of water weights, which are foam barbells that create resistance under water.

1. Get into the swimming pool with your barbells.

2. Stand in the water at about chest level with your arms at your sides as you hold the weights.

3. With your palms facing up, raise your forearms to the water surface, keeping them horizontal to the water. Keep your elbows close to the sides of your body.

4. Turn the barbells over so that your palms are facing the bottom of the pool. Push your hands down until your arms are straight.

5. Repeat 10 to 12 times.

Herbs: Roasted Dandelion Kudzu "Coffee"

Kudzu, a Chinese medicinal herb, can help curb cravings, and dandelion root can help aid in liver detoxification. This beverage is naturally rich and deliciously sweet, with a taste similar to coffee. You can either gather dandelion roots from the ground (they look like weeds) or buy a premade mix (Dandy Blend is a brand I like) at a health food store.

- 1½ teaspoons kudzu powder
- 2 cups water, plus 2 tablespoons
- 1 to 2 teaspoons roasted dandelion root powder
- Pinch of sea salt

1. Dissolve the kudzu powder in 2 tablespoons of water and set aside.

2. Combine the dandelion root powder and 2 cups of water in a pan and simmer for 10 minutes.

3. Add the sea salt and kudzu mixture.

4. Continue simmering for another minute until the mixture thickens.

5. Drink as is or with a splash of milk.

Optional: You can turn this into a creamy, frothy latte by adding in a nut milk of your choice (e.g., oat or almond milk). Drizzle in a sweetener of your choice and blend to create a smooth, frothy latte.

Continued >

Herbs: Roasted Dandelion Kudzu "Coffee" continued

Tip: Did you know you can make your own dandelion root powder? Here's how.

1. *Wash and dry the dandelion roots.*
2. *Mince and spread them on a roasting pan. Bake at 200°F for 4 to 5 hours until completely dry.*
3. *Allow them to cool.*
4. *Grind them into a powder (you can use a coffee grinder).*

ALLERGIES

Allergies can cause symptoms such as skin irritation, hives, sneezing, runny nose, and diarrhea, and they can be triggered by foods, pollen, mold, chemicals, and environmental pollutants. Fortunately, you can use natural treatments such as nettle, raw honey, and bee pollen to help reduce symptoms and avoid the side effects of allergy medication.

Herbs: Nettle Infusion

Nettle leaf is a natural antihistamine, found in most health food stores. It reduces the body's ability to produce histamine, a chemical created by the body to fight against allergens. Stinging nettle's green leaves can fight against those annoying allergy symptoms like runny noses, sneezing, watery eyes, and coughing.

To make a hot herbal tea infusion, you need to buy loose-leaf tea. Hot herbal tea infusions use a larger amount of herbs and are steeped for several hours so the vitamins and enzymes are fully drawn out. The longer the tea is steeped, the more nutrients it provides.

- 3 tablespoons dried stinging nettle
- 1 quart water

Continued >

Herbs: Nettle Infusion continued

1. Place the nettle in a mason jar.

2. Boil the water, then fill the jar to the top with the water. Cover with a lid.

3. Let the tea steep for at least 1 hour. (To maximize the extraction of minerals from the nettles, steep longer—up to 24 hours.)

4. Strain and drink right away or store in the refrigerator for up to 3 days. You can re-steep the tea by adding more water to the mason jar.

Tip: The more nettles you use, the stronger the tea will taste and the more nutrients it will provide. While nettle itself has a mild taste, you can play around with flavors by adding the following: lemon juice, sage leaves, orange peel, or mint leaves. You can also sweeten the infusion with 1 teaspoon of local raw honey.

Herbs: Elderflower Tea

Drinking medicinal tea can be a useful ritual to incorporate into your healing routine. Elderflower is the white blossom of the elderberry tree. This flower has amazing anti-inflammatory and antiseptic properties that can calm the nerves and heal problems with the sinuses, eyes, lungs, and respiratory system. It's commonly used for colds and flu, sinus infections, and other respiratory issues. This herb can be very effective at alleviating allergy symptoms and boosting the immune system. Its delicate flavor also combines nicely with other herbs.

- 2 cups water
- 2 teaspoons dried elderflower

1. Bring the water to a boil.
2. Drop the elderflower into the boiling water and remove from the heat.
3. Allow the elderflower to brew in the water for 5 to 10 minutes. The longer it steeps, the stronger and more potent your tea will be.
4. Drink it warm, or add ice to make iced tea.

Herbs: Pineapple-Turmeric Juice

Bromelain is an enzyme found in the core and flesh of pineapples. It is a natural remedy for inflammation and can help reduce allergies thanks to its anti-inflammatory and anti-allergic properties. Quercetin is a natural antioxidant and antihistamine and can be very helpful in relieving allergy symptoms. It's a natural compound found in plant food such as citrus fruits, turmeric, apples, cranberries, dark berries, kale, and watercress. Its anti-inflammatory

Continued >

REMEDIES

properties can help reduce redness and itchy eyes. This juice makes two servings, so drink one immediately and store the other in a large mason jar for up to two days in the refrigerator.

- 1 pineapple
- 2 oranges
- 1 apple
- 1 lemon
- 1 (2-inch) piece unpeeled turmeric root (or 1 tablespoon turmeric powder)
- 1 to 2 tablespoons raw honey, to taste

1. Cut and slice the pineapple, oranges, apple, and lemon.

2. Run the fruits through a juicer to extract the juice.

3. Run the turmeric root through the juicer.

4. Add the raw honey to the juice and gently stir.

5. Drink one serving immediately, then refrigerate the rest of the juice for up to 2 days.

Tip: You can also take quercetin supplements of 300 to 500 milligrams twice per day at the start of allergy season.

ANXIETY

Stress is a common malady that can have profound effects on mental health. Experiencing anxiety or feeling worried is a normal response to the common stresses we face in life, but when it becomes prolonged, issues can arise.

Essential Oils: Diffuse Anxiety Away

Essential oils can be a great support for anxiety since their numerous therapeutic benefits work holistically to soothe and calm emotions, ease tension, and balance moods, creating an enhanced sense of well-being. Using essential oils in a diffuser can create a reassuring and calm environment.

- 5 drops lemon balm essential oil
- 3 drops lemon essential oil
- 3 drops frankincense essential oil

Simply add all the drops of oil into a diffuser to create a peaceful, aromatic environment.

Massage Therapy: Self-Massage for Anxiety

Self-massage can have therapeutic effects to calm your mind and emotions. This is optional, but you can enhance

Continued >

REMEDIES

the effectiveness of the massage by adding in essential oils. Choose a citrus essential oil, such as orange or mandarin, or ylang-ylang, rose, lavender, or neroli.

1. Take a deep breath in through your nose, then a long exhale.

2. Notice where in your body you feel anxiety. What does it look like? What does it feel like? Is it hard or soft? What color is it? See if you can start to change its features. For example, if it's hard as rock, can you soften it?

3. As you exhale, allow the anxiety to dissipate or flow away from you.

4. Roll your shoulders three times.

5. Take your thumb and forefinger and massage your neck along the trapezius (the large muscles that extend over the back of the neck and shoulders).

6. Continue taking deep breaths and exhaling slowly as you massage both shoulders.

7. As you release your breath, it can help if you say *ahhh* or even smile.

8. Now massage your face, near the temples, and work down toward your jaw. Gently work up toward your scalp. Make sure that you are lifting the skin up as you engage the tissue and not just rubbing over the skin.

9. Massage your ears.

10. End the massage by gently shaking your arms and body and rolling your neck around.

Guided Imagery: Visualization Practice

Guided imagery visualizations are a great way to calm anxiety! It is simply a technique that helps the body enter a relaxed state. The easiest way to do this is to close your eyes and imagine the sights and sounds of a place that you find relaxing. Keep in mind that it isn't the type of scene that's important but rather that you use your imagination and senses to transport you to your imagined place.

Imagery can help with anxiety by allowing you to visualize and focus on positive outcomes rather than negative emotions.

1. Sit or lie down comfortably.
2. Take a deep breath from your diaphragm and count to three as you inhale. Feel your stomach rise as you breathe in.
3. Hold your breath for three seconds.
4. Slowly exhale for a count of three.
5. Repeat until you feel relaxed. (Don't worry if you don't get it right the first time. Deep breathing is a learned skill that requires practice.)

Continued >

Guided Imagery: Visualization Practice continued

6. Next, visualize yourself walking along a white, sandy beach. Imagine the white sand and blue sky. Picture the clear waves crashing gently along the beach. Continue to keep your eyes closed, keeping this beautiful and serene scene in mind. Hear the sound of the waves gently rolling onto the shore. Feel the water touch your bare feet. Feel the warm sand underneath your feet and the warm rays of sunshine on your face. What are your other senses doing? Are you drinking something? What does it taste like? Use all your senses as you continue to imagine and feel yourself in this scene. Notice how calm and relaxed you feel.

7. When you are ready, open your eyes and return to your present surroundings. You should now be alert, and a calm state should have replaced any feelings of anxiety you had. The key is to hold on to this feeling of calmness and use it throughout the day.

ARTHRITIS

The word "arthritis" comes from the Greek word *arthro*, meaning "joint," and the suffix "-itis," meaning "inflammation." A more severe form of arthritis, rheumatoid arthritis (RA), is a chronic autoimmune disease that affects the joints and causes pain, swelling, and stiffness in the limbs. The underlying cause of RA is inflammation, and the sooner you receive treatment for it, the better you'll feel.

If you take a holistic approach to managing RA symptoms by eating an anti-inflammatory diet, staying active, and exploring methods to reduce the pain naturally, you can help improve the quality of your life and prevent further joint damage.

Herbs: Turmeric Paste and Golden Milk

This is a classic Ayurveda turmeric paste that can be used to make golden milk, a warm, healing beverage with anti-inflammatory and antioxidant benefits. Golden milk originated in India and has been used to support the body and mind. In today's busy world, creating this recipe may take a bit of time. So, it's a good idea to make the paste in advance; it will save time later on. You can also purchase the paste at a health food store or online. It's traditionally

Continued >

REMEDIES

made by mixing turmeric and ghee, and it can be stored in the refrigerator until you're ready to make the golden milk.

Turmeric can help reduce pain and swelling in arthritis patients. This recipe is boosted with additional medicinal spices that also have anti-inflammatory properties. Cloves contain eugenol, an anti-inflammatory chemical that interferes with the process that triggers arthritis pain.

For the turmeric paste
- ½ cup organic turmeric powder
- 1 to 1½ cups filtered water
- ¼ teaspoon black pepper
- 2 teaspoons cinnamon powder
- 2 teaspoons cardamom powder
- 1½ teaspoons ginger powder
- ½ teaspoon clove powder
- 1 teaspoon nutmeg powder
- Pinch of Himalayan sea salt
- ½ cup ghee (or coconut oil as a vegan option)

For the golden milk
- 1 cup coconut milk or any nut milk of choice
- 1 to 2 teaspoons turmeric paste
- Yacon syrup, raw honey, coconut sugar, liquid stevia, or other healthy sweetener of choice

To make the turmeric paste

1. Put the turmeric powder and water in a saucepan over medium-low heat, stirring constantly. Keep stirring for a few minutes until the mixture has reached a paste-like consistency. (Use more or less water depending on how thick or thin a consistency you prefer.)

2. Slowly stir in the pepper, cinnamon, cardamom, ginger, clove, nutmeg, and salt.

3. Add the ghee and mix thoroughly.

4. While the paste is still warm and runny, pour it into a glass container. Let it cool, and then refrigerate. The mixture will thicken as it cools. It may be stored in the refrigerator for up to 3 weeks.

To make the golden milk

1. In a small pot, gently heat the milk over low heat until it's warm but not hot.

2. Add 1 or 2 teaspoons of the turmeric paste to the warmed milk.

3. Add your desired sweetener.

Essential Oils: Pain-Relief Blend

Essential oils are often used for their mild anesthetic properties, which can help relieve localized pain. Oils such as rose, eucalyptus, clove, and bergamot can work on the body in a similar way to nonsteroidal anti-inflammatory drugs, such as ibuprofen, by inhibiting the enzymes in the body that cause inflammation, pain, and swelling.

- 2 drops cypress essential oil
- 2 drops sweet marjoram essential oil
- 2 drops ylang-ylang essential oil
- 2 drops peppermint essential oil
- 2 drops black pepper essential oil
- 2 drops ginger essential oil
- 10 ml glass bottle filled with almond oil, coconut oil, or other carrier oil of choice

1. Add all the essential oils to the bottle of almond oil or other carrier oil. Shake the bottle well.
2. Apply a few drops and massage into your skin to relieve pain.

Tip: Taking a hot shower or bath before applying the oils will increase blood flow and enhance their effect. Also, applying the oils just before bed can be helpful for promoting restful sleep as well as supporting deep healing and recovery.

Meditation: Kundalini Meditation

Many cases of chronic pain in conditions like RA can be exacerbated by emotional stress and tension in the body. Pain is magnified when coupled with negative emotions such as anger, frustration, fear, hopelessness, jealousy, or sadness. Regular meditation may help ease arthritis symptoms by helping you to stop focusing on the pain and to break negative thinking patterns.

This is an example of a simple meditation technique that you can start off with, whether you're on the go or sitting quietly.

1. Lie down in a comfortable place. It can be a yoga mat, a couch, or a bed.

2. Close your eyes and turn your focus to your breath. Breathe deeply in through your nose and slowly out through your mouth. As you breathe in, imagine your breath circulating throughout your body to your arms, legs, and stomach. As you exhale, imagine your breath leaving those areas, taking toxins with it. Repeat this for several breaths.

3. Visualize a green light coming into your body. Feel this light penetrating every part of your body. Allow the light to touch on the area that is in pain or needs healing. Imagine this green light touching every cell in that part of your body and restoring it back to health.

4. Take a deep breath in and hold it. Deeply exhale.

ASTHMA

Asthma is a chronic lung disease that affects many people of all ages. The airways that carry oxygen in and out of the lungs become irritated and inflamed, causing the muscles surrounding the airway to tighten and mucus to build up. Many people with asthma have difficulty breathing and frequently wheeze and/or cough. Here are some holistic remedies that can help ease the restrictions caused by asthma.

Essential Oil: Homemade Vapor Rub

Over-the-counter vapor rub is used on the chest and throat to relieve congestion. However, these rubs often contain ingredients that are not healthy and don't address the source of the problem. You can make this simple but effective six-ingredient vapor rub at home. Eucalyptus can help with sinus and respiratory problems, and frankincense can be used to reduce inflammation. These essential oils increase airflow and help relieve congestion.

- ¼ cup beeswax pellets
- ¼ cup olive oil
- ½ cup coconut oil
- 20 drops peppermint essential oil
- 20 drops eucalyptus essential oil
- 10 drops frankincense essential oil

1. Place the beeswax pellets in a glass jar and pour the olive oil and coconut oil over them.

2. Add 2 inches of water to a saucepan and warm over medium-low heat.

3. Put the glass jar in the saucepan, allowing the oils to melt. Stir to combine.

4. Remove the pan from the heat and allow the mixture to cool slightly. Then add the peppermint, eucalyptus, and frankincense essential oils.

5. Pour the mixture into metal tins or storage containers and allow to set.

6. Rub the mixture over the chest or back as needed to relieve congestion.

Breath Work: 4-7-8 Breathing

One of the ways that we can connect with the life force is through our breath. By altering the rhythm of our breathing, we can have a powerful effect on our emotions and physical condition. It's one of the best and easiest tools to combat the effects of stress, asthma, allergies, and just about any ailment.

Breathing may be a natural activity, but some people are not doing it correctly. Often, they are breathing short,

Continued >

Breath Work: 4-7-8 Breathing continued

shallow breaths with their chest. According to Mark Courtney, a therapist with the American Lung Association, it's important to learn to breathe correctly, especially if you have asthma. Breathing through the nose and from the belly can help.

It helps to put one hand on your heart and the other hand on your belly. As you inhale, breathe deeply into your belly; don't suck it in. Instead, let it rise up. When you exhale, bring your belly back in toward your spine.

The 4-7-8 breathing exercise, also known as Relaxing Breath, is simple and can be done anywhere. It will help calm you and relieve stress.

1. Sit comfortably.

2. Place the tip of your tongue against the soft area just behind your upper front teeth and keep it there as you perform the breathing exercise.

3. Keeping your mouth closed, inhale through your nose for a count of four.

4. Hold your breath for a count of seven.

5. Slightly open your mouth and exhale for a count of eight.

Food: Breathe Easy Syrup

This simple syrup can help break up congestion and open up the breathing passages. When you feel an asthmatic episode coming on, take 1 teaspoon of this syrup.

- ½ cup raw honey
- ½ cup fresh lemon juice
- 1 (1-inch) piece ginger root
- 6 garlic cloves
- ¼ teaspoon cayenne pepper

1. Put all the ingredients into a blender or food processor and blend. Pour into a mason jar or other glass jar.
2. Store at room temperature for up to 2 days or in the refrigerator for up to 1 week.

BACK PAIN

Back pain is a very common condition and can make it difficult to function effectively. Whether it's persistent lower back pain, back spasms, or chronic back pain, the common root cause is often inflammation. Eating foods and taking herbs or supplements that lower inflammation can relieve the pain or tension in your back. Fortunately, there are many home-based alternative treatments for back pain.

Essential Oils: First Chakra Oil Blend

According to Ayurveda teachings, the first chakra (the root chakra or *muladhara*) is located at the end of the tailbone, and its role focuses on security and survival. Its function is to support healthy skeletal and nervous systems. Signs of a blocked first chakra include sciatica and skeletal imbalances. Sciatica is characterized by a shooting pain that usually radiates from the lower back down to one leg.

Helichrysum is an essential oil with anti-inflammatory, mild sedative, and analgesic properties. This oil can be one of the fastest acting forms of pain relief compared to most other oils. Eucalyptus has a warm and soothing effect on muscles and can help improve circulation. Ginger is also a warming herb known to ease pain.

Essential oils are very concentrated so it is recommended to dilute them in a carrier oil such as fractionated coconut oil or almond oil. They're also sensitive to heat and light, so be sure to use a dark-colored glass bottle. Many roller bottles are made with thick, anti-shock glass that's resistant to corrosion and amber, which protects against UV rays. For this recipe, you can use the 10-milliliter roller bottle.

Blend #1
- 10 ml fractionated coconut oil
- 2 drops helichrysum essential oil
- 2 drops myrrh essential oil
- 5 drops patchouli essential oil
- 7 drops vetiver essential oil
- 7 drops ylang-ylang essential oil

Blend #2
- 10 ml fractionated coconut oil
- 2 drops cypress essential oil
- 2 drops ylang-ylang essential oil
- 2 drops eucalyptus essential oil
- 3 drops ginger essential oil

1. Fill a 10-milliliter dark roller bottle with the fractionated coconut oil. Add the essential oils from either blend and shake to combine.

Continued >

Essential Oils: First Chakra Oil Blend continued

2. Apply a few drops of this blend to the area where your first chakra is. Massage it in to relieve pain. Alternatively, apply this blend to a warm compress or diffuser.

Tip: Taking a hot shower or Epsom salt bath before applying this oil blend will increase blood flow and enhance the results. Applying it just before bed can promote deep and restful sleep, which also supports recovery.

Food: Ginger, Turmeric, and Cherry Tonic

Ginger and turmeric are a dynamic combination for fighting pain in the body. Turmeric can reduce inflammation, while ginger can stimulate circulation, bringing warmth to the extremities.

- 1 tea bag black tea
- ¼ teaspoon ground ginger
- ¼ teaspoon ground turmeric
- 2 ounces tart cherry juice

1. Place the tea bag in a mug. Add the turmeric and ginger.
2. Fill the mug with boiling water.
3. Cover and steep for 3 to 5 minutes.

4. Add the cherry juice to the mug.

5. Remove the tea bag and enjoy.

Hydrotherapy: Epsom Salt and Lavender Bath

The lavender oil in this mixture can help improve circulation, and the magnesium content in Epsom salt can help restore muscles.

- 1 cup Epsom salt
- 2 drops lavender essential oil

1. Draw a warm bath.

2. Add the Epsom salt and the lavender essential oil.

Tip: For variety, try substituting eucalyptus, clove, or wintergreen essential oil.

COLD AND FLU

A sore throat, runny nose, congested head, and general sense of feeling unwell all signal the start of a cold. The flu virus, which attacks the respiratory system, can be more complicated and severe. Flu is usually accompanied by fever and can produce sweats, chills, and muscle aches. The following home remedies are effective at reducing the symptoms and duration of colds and the seasonal flu.

Herbs: Elderberry Syrup

Elderberry syrup is very easy to make and can help fight the common cold and flu. The dark purple elderberry is known for having powerful natural antiviral effects that can help lessen the symptoms of the cold and flu. This recipe also contains clove and raw honey, which contain antioxidants and natural antiviral and antifungal properties. Adults can take 1 tablespoon daily; children can take 1 teaspoon daily.

- 1 cup dried elderberries
- 4 cups filtered water
- 1 cinnamon stick
- 1 (2-inch) piece ginger, peeled
- 1 teaspoon dried cloves
- 1 cup raw honey

1. Add the elderberries, water, cinnamon stick, ginger, and cloves to a large pot and bring to a boil over medium heat.

2. Reduce the heat to low and continue to simmer for 45 minutes.

3. Remove the pot from the heat and allow the liquid to cool completely.

4. Strain the elderberry mixture using a cheesecloth or a nut bag.

5. Add the raw honey and whisk gently to combine. (Make sure the liquid has completely cooled so the heat doesn't kill off the beneficial enzymes in the raw honey.)

Tips: At the first sign of illness, increase the dosage to every 2 to 3 hours for both adults and children. If you prefer, you can substitute 1 teaspoon of dried ginger or 1 drop of ginger essential oil for the fresh ginger. You can also substitute 1 drop of clove essential oil for the dried cloves. Store the syrup in an airtight glass container and refrigerate for up to 2 months.

Remedies for Health and Healing   115

Herbs: Yarrow and Chamomile Tea

This is a tea you can make if you have a cold or flu accompanied by a fever. Yarrow is thought to have both anti-inflammatory and antimicrobial properties. In ancient times, it was called *herbe militaris*, or the military herb, because it was often used to halt bleeding and heal wounds. Both yarrow and elderflower are considered diaphoretic—in herbalism this means they induce sweating by gently raising body temperature.

Chamomile is a classic herb that promotes relaxation and deep sleep. Yarrow does have a slightly bitter taste, which can be masked by adding raw honey and lemon—both of which have the added benefit of being natural cough suppressants.

- 1 teaspoon dried yarrow flower
- 1 teaspoon chamomile
- 1 teaspoon elderflower (optional)
- 3 to 4 peppermint leaves (optional)
- 1 cup hot water
- 1 teaspoon raw honey
- Squeeze of lemon juice (optional)

1. Place the yarrow and chamomile in a French press. (Include the elderflower and peppermint if you wish.)

2. Pour the hot water into the French press.

3. Cover and steep for 30 minutes.

4. Sweeten with raw honey, add the lemon juice (if using), and enjoy.

Food: Grandma's Healing Bone Broth

This homemade bone broth is easy to make from scratch. It's a good idea to whip up a large batch and store a few servings in the freezer. Then, if you start to feel symptoms of the flu or cold coming on, you'll have this tasty remedy ready to enjoy—and to accelerate your healing!

- 1 to 2 large chicken carcasses (or a mix of back-bones and chicken feet)
- 2 celery stalks, chopped
- 2 carrots, chopped
- 1 onion
- 1 (2-inch) piece ginger
- 4 to 5 garlic cloves
- 12 to 14 cups filtered water (enough to cover the ingredients)
- 1 tablespoon apple cider vinegar
- 1 to 2 teaspoons sea salt
- Herbs of choice: thyme, rosemary, parsley, bay leaves

Continued >

Food: Grandma's Healing Bone Broth continued

1. Place the chicken parts, celery, carrots, onion, ginger, and garlic in a large slow cooker and fill with water. Add the vinegar, salt, and herbs.

2. Set the temperature to low, and let it simmer for 12 to 24 hours.

3. Strain the broth through a colander.

4. Pour the broth into mason jars and store in the refrigerator for up to 1 week or in the freezer for a few months.

Tip: If you don't have a slow cooker, you can use a large pot and set the heat to low so the broth simmers gently. You can also use a pressure cooker and fill the water to the max fill line. Select "manual" and pressure cook on high for 120 minutes. Allow the pressure to release naturally. The longer you let the bones simmer, the more nutrients can be extracted from the bone. You can drink the broth as early as 4 hours but, ideally, cook for at least 6 hours to get a more rich and nutrient-dense broth.

CONSTIPATION

Constipation is defined as having bowel movements fewer than three times a week and passing hard, dry stools. Symptoms can include pain, bloating, and straining. Taking laxatives is not a solution to constipation because it does not attack the root of the problem, which can lie in your overall lifestyle. Lifestyle changes that can ease constipation include drinking sufficient liquids and eating plenty of fiber-rich foods every day. Daily movement can also simulate muscle contractions in the colon.

If you suffer from chronic constipation, take heart in the fact that there is relief. It can often be managed effectively with lifestyle changes, diet, and a few natural home remedies. Typical causes of constipation include dehydration, lack of fiber, imbalance of the intestinal flora, stress, nutritional deficiencies, sluggish liver, and certain medications.

Food: Move-It Smoothie

Dark green leafy vegetables are the highlight of this delicious smoothie. These vegetables contain fiber and magnesium, which help keep things moving along. Baby kale has a lighter taste than regular kale. Feel free to swap it out for milder-tasting leafy vegetables such as spinach or

Continued >

Food: Move-It Smoothie continued

Swiss chard. Flaxseeds make a wonderful addition to this smoothie, with 5 grams of added fiber.

- 2 cups coconut water
- 2 cups baby kale or spinach
- ½ avocado
- 2 cups mango
- ½ lemon, juiced
- 1 tablespoon flaxseeds or pumpkin seeds

1. Place the coconut water in a high-speed blender.
2. Add the kale, avocado, mango, lemon juice, and flaxseeds.
3. Blend together until smooth.

Vitamins: Magnesium Drink

Magnesium is an essential mineral and electrolyte that supports the normal function of the body's cells and organs. While there are many forms of magnesium supplements available, magnesium glycinate or magnesium oxide are easier to absorb and can provide a gentle laxative effect. You can find magnesium supplements in powdered or capsule forms. It is recommended that you start off with a small amount of magnesium at a time and take it in between meals for better absorption.

Consult your doctor before taking magnesium if you are pregnant or nursing or before giving to children under four years old.

1. Scoop a serving size of magnesium powder into a cup. Add 3 to 4 ounces of warm water, and stir until it is dissolved.

2. Fill the remainder of the cup with more water and drink immediately.

Massage: Abdominal Massage

Abdominal massage can relieve constipation by stimulating the contractions needed for bowel movement. It is an effective technique with no side effects. Incorporating deep breathing can also help when you try this self-massage for constipation relief. You can also use peppermint oil (in a carrier oil) to stimulate digestion.

Technique #1

1. Lie down on your back in a comfortable place.

2. Start on the lower right-hand side of your stomach and use your fingers to rub in a clockwise circular motion, working your way around the entire abdominal area.

Continued >

Massage: Abdominal Massage continued

3. Gradually move up the length of the colon and across the left side of the hip. Massage down the descending colon.

4. Do this several times.

Technique #2

Press a tennis ball gently into the belly as you move it along the course of the colon. Do this three times, then move it in a clockwise direction three times.

CROHN'S DISEASE

Crohn's disease is an autoimmune disease that causes inflammation of the digestive tract, which can lead to severe abdominal pain, diarrhea, and extreme weight loss. Stress can worsen symptoms for people with Crohn's disease. Conventional drugs are typically prescribed, but they don't always address the underlying problem or promote healing of the digestive track.

Alternative therapies such as biofeedback, hypnotherapy, and guided imagery—which focus on the mind-body connection—can be very helpful for healing the gut. Probiotics can also be beneficial. The goal is to support healthy gut bacteria, reduce inflammation, and encourage healing of the intestinal wall. While there may be no cure for Crohn's disease, there are effective ways to manage symptoms by taking a holistic approach using natural foods and herbs.

Probiotics: Gut-Loving Piña Colada Kefir

Kefir is a fermented drink packed with living probiotics and enzymes that goes through a natural fermentation process. This delicious probiotic drink is sweet and tangy with a little fizz.

Continued >

Probiotics: Gut-Loving Piña Colada Kefir continued

- 2 to 4 tablespoons probiotic coconut water
  (Inner-ēco or other brand of your choice)
- ½ cup aloe vera
- ½ cup pineapple juice
- Juice of 1 lemon
- ½ teaspoon ginger powder
- 2 teaspoons apple cider vinegar
- ½ cup water

Combine all ingredients in a glass jar. Shake well.

Tip: This concoction can be stored in the refrigerator for up to three days. Drink half a cup each day for maximum benefits.

Meditation: Kundalini Meditation

A huge part of healing an autoimmune disease is addressing emotional and spiritual health. Research shows that practicing meditation will lower cortisol, increase gamma-aminobutyric acid (GABA) production, and shift your nervous system into parasympathetic mode.

Cortisol is the inflammation hormone that gets released when you are stressed, while GABA is a neurotransmitter that blocks certain brain signals, producing a calming effect. You can practice any type of meditation as long as you are consistent. Feel free to try the simple active meditation in the Arthritis section (page 105), or you can try this kundalini meditation method.

1. Sit comfortably with your eyes closed.
2. Touch your thumb to your index finger. Say the mantra "Peace."
3. Touch your thumb to your middle finger. Say the mantra "Begins."
4. Touch your thumb to your ring finger. Say the mantra "With."
5. Touch your thumb to your pinky finger. Say the mantra "Me."

Tip: You can go at your own speed, as fast or as slow as you like.

Breathing: Mindful Breathing

Mindful breathing is simply paying attention to the breath exactly as it is. While breathing is a natural process, it also has nourishing powers. Mindful breathing soothes and heals the mind, body, and spirit.

You can practice this exercise anywhere! It need not be reserved just for meditation or yoga sessions. Practice while you're waiting in line at the supermarket, sitting in

Continued >

Breathing: Mindful Breathing continued

a meeting room at work, or getting ready for bed. When we breathe mindfully, our natural relaxation response is engaged, decreasing the production of the stress hormone cortisol in our bodies.

1. Get comfortable. You can either sit up or lie down. Make sure your back is straight and your body is relaxed. Pay attention to your shoulders and forehead.

2. Close your eyes. Take a moment to ground yourself in your present environment, taking note of the space you are in. What does the air feel like?

3. Pay attention to your natural breathing. What is the rhythm like? Don't try to control or change it, just observe it exactly as it moves in the present moment. What do you notice about the pace of your breathing? How deep or shallow is it? Again, don't try to change it.

4. Simply focus on each breath as you inhale and exhale. Observe the pause in between each inhale and exhale.

DEPRESSION

Depression is a common mental disorder experienced by many people at one time or another. It brings symptoms of sadness, loss of interest in activities that used to bring pleasure, changes in appetite, inability to sleep, poor concentration, and even fatigue. Mild to moderate depression can often be successfully managed with a holistic approach. This includes dietary changes, supplements, herbs, massage, movement, natural sunlight, and approaches such as music therapy. A balanced diet and exercise are the key holistic remedies for treating feelings of depression. Avoiding certain foods in excess, like sugar and caffeine, can also help. Getting adequate sunlight is also effective in preventing the blues.

In Traditional Chinese Medicine, liver stagnation is thought to be at the core of depression. A healthy liver is needed to maintain blood sugar levels, filter blood, and remove waste products. If the liver is impaired, the filtration process gets blocked, which causes toxins to circulate the body and affect the brain.

Breath Work: Deep Pranayama

There are many ways of treating depression, and one of them is to use your own breath. By controlling your breath, you can alter your state of mind. Your breath can be a powerful way of coping with temporary emotional states or mild depression.

Pranayama is the practice of breath control in yoga. It involves deep, intentional, effective breathing that calms the mind and the body. For beginners, pranayama starts with simply watching and paying attention to your breathing.

1. Settle into a comfortable position and allow your breathing to slow down.

2. Next, inhale and count how long it takes to take a full breath.

3. Now, breathe out for the same amount of time that you just inhaled.

4. Continue to do this for one minute, balancing the length of the inhalations and exhalations.

5. Then, gradually add another count to each inhalation and each exhalation until you reach a length of time that feels comfortable.

Tip: Before you start, have a goal in mind for how long you'd like to practice, but be ready to shorten that by a few minutes if you feel your depression lifting. You can continue on past your goal for a few minutes if you feel you need to.

Herbs: Uplifting Tea

Certain herbs, such as St. John's wort and gingko biloba, can boost your mood. Another example is Siberian ginseng, which has been used in Eastern countries for centuries to help decrease cortisol levels and reduce depression. It is used to restore the balance of qi and restore vigor by stimulating a healthy appetite and enhancing overall health.

You can buy these herbs at a health food store. In addition, try making a daily ritual of sipping on this herb-infused tea. The simple act of preparing and slowly sipping on warm tea can also be therapeutic.

- 1 tablespoon dried St. John's wort
- 1 tablespoon lemon balm
- 1 tablespoon oatstraw
- ½ tablespoon chamomile

1. Place all the ingredients in a French press, then fill the press with hot water.

2. Steep the mixture for 10 to 15 minutes, or up to 3 hours for a stronger infusion.

3. Pour the tea into a cup and drink.

4. Save the remainder of the tea in the refrigerator for up to 3 days.

REMEDIES

Essential Oils: Good Mood Blend

Essential oils, when diluted in a carrier oil such as fraction-ated coconut oil, can be massaged into the skin and then absorbed into the bloodstream. The following essential oils can be effective in the treatment of depression.

- 2 drops clary sage essential oil
- 2 drops rose essential oil
- 2 drops basil essential oil
- 2 drops lavender essential oil
- 2 drops ylang-ylang essential oil

Place the essential oils in a diffuser with the appropriate amount of water and inhale deeply.

GRIEF

Grief is the most difficult of human sufferings; it can leave a person feeling deeply discouraged and despondent. In addition to the emotional pain it can cause, there are often physical manifestations as well. When you are grieving, your heart rate and adrenaline production can increase. It is not unusual to experience chest pain or a sensation of numbness in your limbs. In Chinese medicine, the lungs and heart are thought to be associated with grief. A heavy heart that lasts for an extended time can also lead to a weakened immune system and illness. Recovering from grief is difficult, but you can support your body during this time with these holistic remedies.

Energy Healing: Revitalizing Energy Exercise

One form of natural healing for grief is energy healing, which can change your energy from negative to positive, from depressed to feeling uplifted. All emotions are some form of energy. Holistic healers believe that when you feel grief, you are experiencing a real emotional energy in your body. When you are deeply sad, you probably notice a heavy feeling in your chest. An energy healer can work with you to send energy into this area that has been

Continued >

Energy Healing: Revitalizing Energy Exercise continued

disconnected from life-force energies. Like all emotions, grief is meant to move through a person, not get stuck in the physical body.

There are many forms of energy healing. You can work with a Reiki practitioner in your area or try this DIY technique at home. This technique aims to evoke and release the energies of anger or frustration that can come with grief.

1. Stand up straight.
2. Put your arms out in front of you, with your elbows slightly bent.
3. Make fists with the inside of your wrists facing up.
4. Take a full breath.
5. Swing your arms behind you and up over your head. Pause for a moment.
6. Reach up high, and turn your fists so your fingers are facing each other. Bring your arms down in a swift motion in front of your body, as you release your fists.
7. Let out your breath and emotions with a *whoosh* sound.
8. Repeat two to three times.

Essential Oils: Grief Support Roller Bottle

Essential oils can stimulate chemical changes in brain chemistry by opening different neural pathways. Add some essential oils to a bath and let the tears flow. Crying helps provide emotional release. You can also add the essential oils to a roller bottle and massage over the chest. For this remedy, you'll need 10 milliliters of fractionated coconut oil and two to five of the following essential oils.

- Cedarwood essential oil
- Frankincense essential oil
- Rose essential oil
- Clary sage essential oil
- Geranium essential oil
- Ginger essential oil
- Lavender essential oil
- Lemon balm essential oil
- Jasmine essential oil
- Neroli essential oil
- Petitgrain essential oil

1. Put 2 drops each of the essential oils you have chosen in a 10-milliliter roller bottle.

2. Fill the bottle to the top with fractionated coconut oil.

3. Massage in a circular motion over the heart and lungs.

Flower Essence: Star of Bethlehem Water

Holistic healing often uses flower essence to help those dealing with grief. Many people find that consuming these essences can help foster a sense of comfort and support. Star of Bethlehem is highly beneficial for supporting our ability to move through trauma, loss, and shock by easing feelings of sorrow, sadness, and grief and helping bring a sense of comfort.

1. Put 2 drops of Star of Bethlehem essence in a glass of water.
2. Drink and repeat up to a total of three times a day.

HEADACHES/MIGRAINES

Headaches can be both painful and debilitating. A headache is an SOS message from your body that something is wrong. While there are numerous effective home remedies that can get rid of the temporary pain, it's worth looking into the underlying causes so you can prevent headaches in the future.

Many things can contribute to headaches including deficiency in minerals (such as magnesium), food intolerances, stress, and lack of sleep. If you've suffered from migraines, you know that they are usually more intense and uncomfortable than a typical headache. Migraines can be triggered by many different things including hormonal changes, stress, noises, smells, and certain foods. A diet rich in magnesium may help prevent headaches. Magnesium-rich foods include dark leafy greens, avocados, nuts, seeds, legumes, and even dark chocolate.

Acupressure: Acupressure for Headache Relief

You can do acupressure at home by using two fingers to apply pressure to specific places on your body called acupoints. You can do acupressure several times a day or as often as needed for your symptoms to go away. In order to

Continued >

Acupressure: Acupressure for Headache Relief continued

do it safely, never do acupressure on areas of the skin that have open cuts or swelling.

There's a pressure point known in Traditional Chinese Medicine as *hegu*, which is located between the base of your thumb and index finger. Applying pressure to this point sometimes relieves headache pain.

1. Using your right thumb and index finger, find the space on your left hand between the base of your thumb and index finger.

2. Gently pinch this spot and massage in a circular motion without lifting your thumb and index finger. Do this for five minutes.

3. Repeat the process on your right hand.

Essential Oil: Peppermint Magic Compress

Peppermint essential oil is an excellent natural remedy for headaches. A study in the *Asian Pacific Journal of Tropical Biomedicine* suggests that massaging peppermint oil onto your temples and forehead is as effective at relieving headache pains as over-the-counter medicine such as ibuprofen. Peppermint essential oil contains the active compound menthol, which can help relieve pain.

1. Wet a washcloth with cold water and wring it dry.

2. Put a few drops of peppermint essential oil onto the washcloth to use as a compress.

3. Hold the compress to your head. This can stimulate nerve endings on the face and scalp, which sends signals to the brain that may decrease pain.

Vitamins and Minerals: Mineral-Rich Spa Water

One cause of your headaches could be a mineral deficiency, specifically of magnesium. Magnesium is a powerful mineral that serves many functions in our body, including controlling nerve function and cortisol levels. Adding Himalayan sea salt to your water can help replenish some of the minerals your body is missing. I've included a recipe for making a brine with Himalayan sea salt called sole (pronounced "solay") water. It contains 84 trace minerals. It's important to use a good, high-quality sea salt that is sourced from ancient sea beds rather than standard table salt. A recipe for a delicious Mineral-Rich Spa Water follows.

For the sole water

- ½ cup Himalayan sea salt
- 32 ounces filtered water

Continued >

REMEDIES

For the mineral-rich spa water
- Juice of ½ lemon
- 32 ounces filtered water or coconut water
- ½ tablespoon sole water
- ¼ cup pomegranate, cranberry, or cherry juice
- ¼ cup sliced cucumbers
- 4 to 5 peppermint or spearmint leaves

To make the sole water
1. Put ½ cup Himalayan sea salt in a large mason jar filled with 32 ounces filtered water.
2. Let the mixture sit overnight, or up to 24 hours.
3. In the morning, you will have your sole water (this is your base brine). Sole water can be kept in the refrigerator for up to 3 weeks.

When you have a headache, scoop out 1 tablespoon of that brine and add it to a glass. Add lemon if desired.

To make the mineral-rich spa water
1. Add the lemon juice, filtered water, sole water, pomegranate juice, and cucumber.
2. Bruise the mint leaves by slapping them against your palms to release the natural oils.
3. Add the mint leaves to the water.
4. Drink immediately, with or without ice.

HIGH BLOOD SUGAR

Type 2 diabetes now affects more than 27 million people in America. Controlling blood sugar is critical for someone who has diabetes. The ability of the body to properly control the levels of blood sugar and regulate insulin and cortisol is essential for promoting health and longevity. Sedentary habits and an unhealthy diet particularly high in refined sugar and carbohydrates are two of the major risk factors for the development of type 2 diabetes.

Food: Aloe Green Smoothie

Aloe vera is a medicinal plant that has been used in Traditional Chinese Medicine for over 2,000 years. Aloe vera may help lower blood sugar and manage insulin sensitivity. Insulin is a hormone that allows sugar molecules to enter the body's cells.

This refreshing drink tastes amazing. It's sweetened naturally by coconut water, or you can add yacon syrup or liquid stevia. Yacon syrup has a low glycemic index, which means it is less likely than other sweeteners to raise blood sugar. It tastes similar to molasses and is an excellent substitute for sugar—and a little bit goes a long way! In

Continued >

Food: Aloe Green Smoothie continued

addition, yacon syrup is considered by holistic healers to be medicinal due to its high level of antioxidants.

- 2 cups coconut water
- 1 aloe vera leaf (or 2 ounces aloe vera juice)
- 1 tablespoon green juice powder
- ½ cup ice
- ¼ teaspoon yacon syrup or a few drops of liquid stevia (optional)

Blend ingredients in a high-speed blender and enjoy!

Herbs: Healing Adaptogenic Elixir

There is a category of herbs called adaptogens that are commonly used in Traditional Chinese Medicine and Ayurveda. Adaptogens may help regulate blood sugar by reducing elevated cortisol and blood sugar levels. Helpful adaptogens include ashwagandha, American ginseng, Asian ginseng, cordyceps, holy basil, reishi, rhodiola, and shilajit.

This creamy and luscious elixir tastes like hot chocolate—but with added benefits!

- 1½ cups organic coconut milk
- 1 tablespoon raw cacao powder
- ½ teaspoon maca powder

- 1 teaspoon chia seeds
- ½ teaspoon cinnamon
- ½ teaspoon reishi
- ½ teaspoon ashwagandha
- ½ teaspoon cordyceps
- Pinch Himalayan sea salt

1. Warm the coconut milk in a small pot. Add the rest of the ingredients.

2. Transfer the mixture to a blender and blend until creamy and frothy.

3. Add an optional low-glycemic sweetener such as 1 to 2 drops of liquid stevia, monkfruit extract, ½ teaspoon of coconut sugar, or yacon syrup. Serve chilled or warm—whichever you prefer!

Tip: This recipe can easily be adapted to your own taste preference. Use a dairy-free milk of choice and adjust the sweetener. If you decide to use hot water in place of milk, add 1 tablespoon of coconut butter for creaminess and additional healthy fats.

Exercise: Yoga Cobra Pose

Any type of movement can be an effective form of treatment for people with type 2 diabetes. The key is to choose something you'll enjoy and look forward to doing every day. Yoga is a great example of an exercise that helps reduce high blood sugar levels and control blood glucose.

It's best to start with at least one initial session taught by a yoga instructor. After that, and as soon as you feel comfortable, you can practice yoga in the comfort of your own home. Many yoga teachers offer classes, CDs, and recordings. Try this basic yoga pose at home!

The cobra pose is one of the foundational poses in yoga and includes mindful breathing. It can improve overall health but more specifically, it helps stimulate and rejuvenate the pancreas (and improve the organ's ability to produce insulin). It should be done on the floor.

1. Lie facedown on your stomach and extend your legs out straight. Bring your feet together with your toes pointing outward. Gently rest your forehead on the floor.

2. Place your palms under your shoulders and as you breathe in, lift up your upper body using your arms for support.

3. Arch your back as far as you can and shift your gaze to the ceiling.

4. Hold this pose for at least a minute. (After you've gotten some practice in, try holding it longer.)

5. Take a deep breath and then lower yourself back to the starting position, exhaling as you do so.

INFERTILITY

Infertility is a challenge that can take a physical and emotional toll on anyone trying to conceive. Combining conventional medicine with holistic aids may give you the best chance at reversing infertility. In addition to the suggested remedies in this section, you should consider removing gluten, dairy, and sugar from your diet, and limiting excess coffee. According to Traditional Chinese Medicine, infertility is an indication of an excess of yin, caused by eating too much dairy and gluten. Also, too much caffeine promotes inflammation and can create an imbalance of hormones. You can also consider supplementing your diet with so-called fertility superfoods such as spirulina, royal jelly, and maca powder, as well as foods that are high in antioxidants.

Herbs: Fertility Energy Protein Bars

Maca is a root vegetable that has been used as an aphrodisiac to boost fertility and sex drive in women and men for centuries. Traditionally, this "Peruvian ginseng" was taken for increased energy and stamina. Maca has also been known to support women's bodies to restore hormonal balance. Adding in ashwagandha can also help increase sperm count for men.

- ¼ cup dates
- ¼ cup dried fruit (apricots, cranberries, or cherries)
- 1 cup almond flour
- ½ cup hemp seeds
- 1 tablespoon maca powder (or ½ tablespoon maca powder plus ½ tablespoon ashwagandha powder)
- ½ teaspoon cinnamon
- ½ tablespoon bee pollen
- ½ cup walnuts
- ½ cup almonds
- ¼ cup raw honey
- ½ teaspoon vanilla extract or vanilla powder

1. Remove the pits from the dates if needed. Chop the dates and dried fruit into small pieces (you can also use a food processor to chop them).

2. Combine the almond flour, hemp seeds, maca powder, cinnamon, bee pollen, dates, dried fruits, walnuts, and almonds in a bowl and mix well.

3. Add the honey and vanilla extract. Mix thoroughly.

4. Transfer the mix to an 8-by-8-inch nonstick pan.

5. Place the pan in the refrigerator for at least 1 hour to allow the mixture to firm up.

6. Cut into bars and enjoy. Store the leftovers in a tightly sealed container for up to 2 weeks.

Herbs: Shatavari Fertility Elixir

Shatavari is one of the best herbs for women's reproductive health. The name actually means "she who possesses 100 husbands." Grown in India, it has been used by Ayurveda healers for hundreds of years as a female tonic. It has no toxic side effects and may help improve overall fertility. The simplest and most traditional way to consume shatavari is by making a paste, a basic Ayurveda method of cooking. Simply combine the powdered herb with a bit of ghee and honey, then add it to milk and drink every day. The healthy fats from ghee aid in the absorption of the herb.

You can also make this creamy elixir, which tastes delicious. The adaptogens in this elixir are specifically aimed at supporting women's reproductive health. Lowering stress is also an important part of a holistic plan for fertility, and these adaptogens are perfect since they can help your body and mind adapt to stressful situations. This drink can be stored in the refrigerator for up to two days.

- 2 cups almond milk or gluten-free oat milk
- 1 teaspoon maca powder
- 1 teaspoon shatavari
- 1 tablespoon cacao powder
- 1 teaspoon ashwagandha powder
- 2 teaspoons tahini
- 2 teaspoons raw honey
- ¼ teaspoon cinnamon

1. Warm the almond milk in a saucepan over low heat.

2. Whisk in the maca, shatavari, cacao, and ashwagandha until thoroughly mixed.

3. Add the tahini and honey, and whisk.

4. Transfer to a blender and blend for 20 seconds for a creamy and frothy drink. Top with cinnamon before serving.

Massage Therapy: Castor Oil

Castor oil therapy has been used for centuries to promote healing in the reproductive system, lymphatic system, and circulatory system. Castor oil can also stimulate detoxification systems in the body, including the lymphatic system and the liver. It's important that you have good circulation so your body can eliminate toxins, dead tissues, and old blood. You can make your own castor oil pack by following these instructions.

- 1 flannel cloth
- Large square container with lid
- 1 bottle castor oil
- Plastic wrap
- Hot water bottle
- Solution of baking soda and water

Continued >

Massage Therapy: Castor Oil continued

1. Place the flannel in the container. Pour the castor oil over the flannel until it is saturated.

2. Place the saturated piece of flannel over your lower abdomen.

3. Wrap your abdomen with plastic wrap, leaving the flannel in place.

4. Place the hot water bottle over the flannel for 30 to 45 minutes.

5. After removing the flannel, cleanse the area with a solution of water and baking soda.

6. Store the flannel in a container, and reuse up to 20 times.

INSOMNIA

Insomnia is a sleep disorder in which a person has trouble falling asleep or achieving a deep sleep. Experiencing an occasional restless night is normal, but chronic sleeplessness can be an indicator of a more serious health issue or an unbalanced lifestyle. Insomnia can affect your hormonal, emotional, and physical health including memory, cognitive ability, and mood.

Throughout the day, your body temperature fluctuates. It reaches the coolest point in the early morning, before waking up. As your body prepares to wake up, cortisol is released, energizing and warming you up. Your body temperature reaches its peak during the day, before cooling down again at night, signaling to your brain that it's time to sleep.

Melatonin, a hormone that our bodies make to help us feel sleepy, is released in the evening. This is triggered by the body's response to reduced light exposure, which happens after the sun goes down. This is also the reason that over-exposure to unnatural light from laptops, televisions, or smart phones inhibits the production of melatonin. Experts recommend that you use blue light–blocking glasses if you plan on using these devices at night. It's also important that you get plenty of natural light during the day. In addition, the following holistic remedies may help you balance your sleep cycles.

REMEDIES

They aim to awaken natural biological rhythms, thereby reducing stress and tension in both the body and mind.

Light Therapy: Natural Sunlight Therapy

Here are a couple of things you can do first thing in the morning to help wake your brain up and regulate your body's natural circadian rhythm.

1. Within an hour of waking up, go outside and face the sunlight. Open your eyes and allow the natural sunlight to hit your face and body. Spend about 30 minutes outside.

2. If you're not able to go outside, turn on a bright light inside. You can also invest in a light therapy lamp that mimics natural sunlight without the harmful UV rays.

Massage Therapy: Abhyanga Massage

Skin care is really a wellness practice because the skin is an organ of communication. It has millions of receptors that are linked to the nervous system and that inform you how to feel and respond. The act of stroking your skin activates your parasympathetic nervous system, which releases oxytocin and produces a calm and relaxed feeling all over.

A warm oil massage is an Ayurvedic practice used to connect with yourself and calm the nervous system. As a bonus, it can also help relax muscles and ease stiff joints in your body. It's one of the ultimate forms of self-care. Abhyanga involves massaging the whole body with a warm Ayurveda herb oil. The practice is very grounding and helps soothe the mind.

- ½ cup sesame oil or coconut oil
- Squeezable bottle
- Pot or pan with hot water
- Large towel

1. Place the oil in the squeeze bottle, then warm it slightly in a pot of hot water over low heat.

2. Sit comfortably on a towel in a warm room.

3. Massage the oil onto your entire body, beginning with your hands. Use your fingers to massage your scalp in any direction. Massage your face in circular movements. Use long strokes to massage your neck.

4. Use long strokes on your arms and circular strokes on your elbows.

Continued >

Massage Therapy: Abhyanga Massage continued

5. Massage your abdomen and chest in broad, clockwise, circular motions. For the armpits and toward the breasts, use long strokes. On the abdomen, move up the right side, then across, then down on the left side. (This also helps with digestion.)

6. Massage the legs using long strokes and the knees using circular strokes.

7. Enjoy a warm bath or shower.

8. When you get out of the bath, towel dry.

9. Put on a pair of cotton socks to protect your environment from the residual oil on your feet.

Tip: In Ayurveda, the medicinal oils used are typically organic, unrefined sesame or coconut oil.

Essential Oils: Sleepy Time Balm

Sleep balms are fun to make, and they only require a few ingredients. Essential oils such as lavender have been known to help people feel relaxed.

- ¼ cup refined coconut oil
- 1 tablespoon beeswax
- 1 teaspoon shea butter or cocoa butter
- 6 drops vetiver essential oil

- 6 drops lavender essential oil
- 6 drops lemon balm essential oil

1. Put the coconut oil, beeswax, and shea butter in a glass bowl, then place the bowl in a pot of hot water, creating a makeshift double boiler.

2. Heat until completely melted. Add the essential oils and pour into small storage containers.

3. Allow the mixture to cool on the countertop.

4. Cover and label the containers when cool.

5. To use, put some balm on your fingers and then massage across the bottom of your feet and along your spine. It may seem greasy at first, but it will be absorbed quickly.

IRRITABLE BOWEL SYNDROME

Irritable bowel syndrome (IBS) is a common gastrointestinal disorder that is believed to be caused by a disconnect between the digestive tract, the brain, and the autonomic nervous system. There is no single identified cause, but it's defined by a cluster of symptoms including frequent abdominal pain or discomfort, bloating, cramps, diarrhea, and constipation. When it comes to IBS, there really isn't one single treatment that will work for everyone. The goal is to manage your lifestyle, as stress and emotions can affect the digestive tract. Along with conventional medicine, there are a range of holistic treatments that may help.

It's not uncommon for people to suffer from IBS for years, since it can be a difficult condition for doctors to diagnose. Conventional doctors often prescribe medication and recommend that patients take in more fiber, but this does not address the underlying causes of IBS. Although the precise causes of IBS are unknown, several factors appear to play a role. These include changes in the bacteria in the gut, abnormal contractions in the intestines, poorly coordinated signals between the brain and the intestines, inflammation of the intestines, and severe infections.

Essential Oils: Peppermint and Ginger Capsule

Peppermint oil can help reduce IBS symptoms by relaxing the smooth muscles in the walls of the intestine. Ginger is another common food often used for gastrointestinal symptoms. Holistic healers use ginger extract as an anti-inflammatory to strengthen the gastric lining and to stimulate motility of the intestines.

The easiest way to take a concentrated amount of peppermint and ginger oil is in a capsule. The oil used in capsules is processed directly from the leaves, stem, and flower of the plant, so you're ingesting more in this form than you would in tea or food. These capsules are enteric, meaning they are encased in a coating that lets them pass through the stomach unaltered and then get released directly into the intestines. This prevents possible indigestion. Peppermint and ginger capsules are available at health food stores and online, or you can make your own, following this recipe.

- Enteric vegetable capsules
- 2 drops ginger essential oil
- 2 drops peppermint oil

1. Carefully put 2 drops each of peppermint essential oil and ginger essential oil in an enteric capsule.
2. Take one capsule with water as needed to aid digestion.

REMEDIES

Meditation: Progressive Muscle Relaxation

Techniques that help reduce nervous system activity and relax muscles are simple and may enhance your healing journey. These include yoga, hypnosis, acupuncture, biofeedback, and herbal remedies.

Your gut and brain have a two-way communication system called the brain-gut axis, consisting of the brain and spinal cord and the enteric nervous system. Did you know that these nerve cells (100 million of them) live in your gastrointestinal tract? This means your brain influences your gut and vice versa. It's a highway of constant communication. Ninety percent of serotonin (a brain neurotransmitter) is produced in the digestive tract and plays a role in bowel movement and function.

This method involves tensing and relaxing your muscles in a sequence that begins at your head and ends at your toes. It may take a bit more effort to do than other techniques, but it can really help manage IBS symptoms.

1. Find a comfortable place to sit or lie down.

2. First, close your eyelids and squeeze them shut while taking a breath and holding for a count of three seconds. Then relax and release the tension.

3. Next tense the muscles in your forehead as if you're frowning. Hold this for three seconds as well.

4. Move down your body, repeating this sequence of tensing and relaxing your muscles. Include your nose,

jaw, face, neck, shoulders, arms, hands, chest, back, abdomen, buttocks, upper legs, lower legs, feet, and finally, your toes.

5. Notice how relaxed your body feels.

6. Now focus on your breath for as long as you wish.

Herbs: Dandelion and Peppermint Tonic

We have things called bitter taste receptors located throughout our gastrointestinal tract, and when they're activated by bitter herbs and foods, they release the saliva, enzymes, and bile we need to break down food. Bitter foods including dandelion and ginger may assist in relieving IBS symptoms.

- 5 to 10 dandelion leaves
- 5 to 10 peppermint leaves
- 1 (2-inch) piece ginger, peeled and thinly sliced

1. Wash the dandelion and peppermint leaves.

2. Slap the peppermint leaves between the palms of your hands to release the natural oils.

3. Gently pound the ginger slices on a cutting board with the back of your knife to release the natural juice.

4. Add the ingredients to a cup of hot filtered water.

Continued >

Herbs: Dandelion and Peppermint Tonic continued

5. Steep for about 10 minutes.

6. Discard the ingredients and drink the tea.

Tip: When you're experiencing digestive dysfunction from IBS or another gut condition, natural processes like enzyme production can lag and further contribute to poor digestion. It might be helpful to take a digestive enzyme supplement before each meal to stimulate digestion.

MEMORY LOSS

Some degree of aging-related memory loss is natural and usually does not affect normal body functions. However, memory loss caused by dementia, such as Alzheimer's disease, can be debilitating. People who suffer from memory loss may benefit from acupuncture or massage therapy. Holistic healing teaches that massage therapy simulates movement and the flow of lymph and blood in the body and that acupuncture can help correct and improve the flow of the body's qi, or life-force energy. Both remedies can give you the gift of touch as well as release the stress and tension caused by memory loss.

Eating a well-balanced diet high in omega-3 fats (such as fish or seeds), beta carotene, folic acid, iron, zinc, and vitamin C can also give your brain a boost. Stimulating your brain by doing mental exercises such as crossword puzzles can also be beneficial.

Nutritional Therapy: Roasted Veggie Chickpea Salad with Blueberry Dressing

The Mediterranean diet includes an abundance of healthy organic fruits and vegetables and healthy fats such as olive oil, nuts, seeds, and wild-caught fish. The keto diet

Continued >

REMEDIES

is another option to explore since it is also high in healthy fats and low in carbohydrates.

This recipe is jam-packed with brain-healthy nutrients like omega-3s from fish oil. Don't worry, some brands (such as Flora Udo's Oil DHA Blend) don't have a fishy smell! The ingredients are nourishing for your brain. You can also add wild-caught salmon for additional healthy fats if you're not a vegetarian.

For the dressing

- ½ cup fresh blueberries
- 3 tablespoons apple cider vinegar
- ½ teaspoon Himalayan sea salt
- ¼ teaspoon black pepper
- 1 teaspoon maple syrup
- ⅓ cup fish oil

For the salad

- 4 medium carrots, peeled and cut into 2-inch pieces
- 4 beets, peeled
- 1 fennel bulb, trimmed and cut into 2-inch pieces
- 1½ tablespoons hemp seed oil or avocado oil
- Pinch Himalayan sea salt
- Pinch black pepper
- ¾ cup chickpeas, cooked
- 4 cups baby arugula, packed

To make the dressing

Blend the blueberries, vinegar, salt, pepper, and maple syrup in a blender on medium-high speed. As the mixture blends, drizzle in the fish oil. Once the dressing is smooth and creamy, taste it and add salt and pepper as needed.

To prepare the salad

1. Preheat the oven to 425°F.

2. Place the carrots, beets, and fennel into a large mixing bowl. Add the oil and toss the vegetables well to coat.

3. Place the coated vegetables onto a lined baking sheet and add a generous sprinkle of coarse salt and black pepper.

4. Roast in the oven for 30 minutes, or until the vegetables are gently browning and tender. Stir once halfway through.

5. To prepare the salad, combine the roasted vegetables with the chickpeas and arugula. Divide the salad onto serving plates and top generously with dressing. Enjoy!

Essential Oils: Diffused Rosemary

Rosemary essential oil may be able to boost memory. All you have to do is breathe it in, especially if you are doing a task that needs focus.

- 4 to 5 drops rosemary essential oil
- Diffuser

Place the rosemary essential oil in a diffuser, and reap the benefits.

Exercise: Hiking

The benefits of exercise are numerous, but did you know that regular exercise may improve memory? A simple walk or hike will do wonders for your brain. You can do this by yourself, or ask a friend to come along.

1. Choose an appropriate trail that is right for your fitness level. Decide on the distance of the trail ahead of time, and make sure the weather is good.

2. Pack a small snack such as nuts, granola bars, or precut fruit. Don't forget to pack a water bottle.

3. Dress comfortably. Wear hiking boots or nonskid shoes.

MUSCLE SPASMS

Muscle spasms are painful involuntary contractions that can occur suddenly throughout the body. They range in intensity from mild twitches to severe pain.

Mineral Therapy: Transdermal Magnesium Massage

Magnesium serves many important functions, including maintaining normal nerve and muscle function. A shortage of magnesium in the body can contribute to muscle spasms. Unfortunately, most people do not meet the daily requirements for magnesium. The easiest remedy is to take a daily magnesium supplement. Alternatively, you can restore your magnesium levels by applying a lotion, gel, or spray to your body.

1. Massage some magnesium lotion or gel directly onto the spasming muscle. It is best to apply it to clean skin.

2. To use a magnesium spray, simply spray two to three times onto the affected muscles and rub until it's fully absorbed.

Yoga: Gentle Asana–Fish Pose

Stretching exercises in yoga are helpful in providing stability and strength for your muscles. Even 15 minutes of stretching every morning or evening can make a world of difference. Asana is a basic term for the many postures in yoga. One of the beginner poses that you can perform to help relieve muscle spasms is the fish pose. This particular pose stretches the front part of the body all the way down to the abdomen and hips. The fish pose can be quite beneficial for treating all kinds of muscle spasms, especially those related to your back and neck.

1. Lie down on your back on a yoga mat or towel.
2. Extend your legs out straight, side by side, and place your arms straight at your sides.
3. Tuck your hands a little bit under your thighs, then with gentle pressure begin to lift your chest upward.
4. Continue lifting up until you reach a position in which you feel comfortable, then hold yourself in this position for three to six deep breaths.
5. Make sure that your head touches the ground throughout this yoga pose.
6. Come back slowly and gradually to your original position.

Acupressure: Acupressure Points Spasms

According to Traditional Chinese Medicine, there are certain acupressure points on your body (acupoints) that can help relieve muscle spasms when pressure is applied. These instructions explain how to activate two different acupoints—the Yang Spring (GB-34) and the Valley of Harmony (LI-4).

To activate the Yang Spring

1. To find this point, start by locating the small knob of bone on the side of your lower right leg (below the knee). Now move your finger to the front and slowly slide it downward. You will find a dip. To activate this acupoint, apply steady pressure with your right thumb until you feel soreness.

2. Hold for three minutes.

3. Repeat on the left leg.

To activate the Valley of Harmony

1. This acupoint—the web between your right thumb and index finger—is believed to affect the upper extremities. To activate this acupoint, apply steady pressure with your left thumb until you feel soreness.

2. Hold for two minutes.

3. Repeat on the left side.

NAUSEA

Nausea can be very uncomfortable and disabling. Common causes of nausea include pregnancy, the side effects of many drugs, motion sickness, and food poisoning. Traditional Chinese Medicine teaches that stomach energy normally flows downward. When it doesn't flow in the right direction, you can experience nausea. This is why it helps to treat the digestive system and stomach to relieve symptoms.

Essential Oil: Personal Nasal Inhaler Bottle with Ginger and Peppermint

This personal nasal inhaler is convenient, as you can carry it in your purse or backpack. Whenever you feel nauseated from motion sickness, car sickness, or any other trigger, simply sniff it. You can buy the personal inhaler online.

- 2 drops peppermint essential oil
- 2 drops ginger essential oil
- 2 drops lemon essential oil
- Personal inhaler with cotton tip absorber

1. Add the essential oils to the cotton part of the nasal inhaler.
2. Inhale deeply through your nose as needed.

3. Add more drops of essential oils to make a stronger combination, but be sure to include equal parts of each.

Tip: As an alternative, you can swap one of the listed oils for orange essential oil.

Acupressure: Deep Breathing with Acupressure

The act of controlled, deep breathing can be incredibly effective for controlling nausea. If you can do this in fresh air, all the better! This controlled breathing technique, in which subjects inhaled through the nose for a count of three, then held their breath for a count of three, then exhaled for a count of three, was shown to reduce nausea by 62 percent!

1. On your left arm, find the acupoint located three finger widths above the wrist crease, between the two tendons on the inside of the left forearm. This is known as acupoint Inner Gate (P-6) in Traditional Chinese Medicine.

2. Apply moderate pressure with your right thumb. Hold for five minutes.

3. Repeat on the right arm.

Food and Herbs: Homemade Ginger Simple Syrup

Ginger root is a popular remedy for a good reason. It really can help alleviate nausea. Ginger has been used for centuries as an aid for nausea treatment, and recent studies have shown that this medicinal root has a strong ability to reduce nausea caused by car sickness, morning sickness for pregnant women, and chemotherapy treatments. Ginger is readily available and many people already have it in the kitchen!

You can either take ginger capsules or make a delicious homemade ginger drink using this ginger simple syrup. Use the syrup to make tea by adding hot water or to make cold ginger ale by adding sparkling mineral water.

- 4 cups filtered water
- 3 knobs of ginger, sliced (about 2 cups)
- ½ cup raw honey
- 1 lemon

1. Bring the filtered water and the ginger to a simmer.

2. Simmer for 20 to 30 minutes.

3. Turn off the heat and allow the mixture to cool.

4. Add the honey.

5. Store the syrup in the refrigerator for up to 1 week.

6. When symptoms arise, add ¼ cup of the ginger mixture to 1 cup sparkling mineral water for ginger ale, or add it to a cup of hot water for ginger tea.

NERVE PAIN

Chronic nerve pain affects more than 50 million Americans, yet management of this pain remains a clinical challenge. Some conventional treatments yield poor results, and patients sometimes suffer from side effects when they take the analgesic medications they are prescribed. Nerve pain can result from injury, illness, nutritional deficiencies, infection, or the side effects from medication. Sometimes it's referred to as neuropathy or peripheral neuropathy, a reference to the peripheral nervous system that sends messages to the brain.

The pain can be characterized as shooting, burning, stabbing, or tingling, as well as numbness in the hands, feet, and back. It can be helpful to complement conventional treatment for nerve pain with some holistic therapies. Herbs, supplements, and essential oils can offer some relief, as can therapies such as yoga and acupuncture.

Acupuncture

Acupuncture can help relieve many of the symptoms of nerve pain, as well as help improve the functioning of the nerves and the body as a whole. According to Traditional Chinese Medicine, the pain and dysfunction resulting from

Continued >

Acupuncture continued

peripheral neuropathy are caused by a blockage of qi energy and blood. It is believed that this prevents cells and tissues from receiving nourishment and can lead to physical problems. The practice of acupuncture helps remove this energy blockage and balance the qi in your body, which enhances the ability of the body to heal. For example, the needles may stimulate the nervous system to release chemicals in the muscles, spinal cord, and brain. Chemicals such as endorphins are considered your body's natural pain killers since they help block the perception of pain.

It is important to receive treatment from an acupuncturist who has met accepted standards for education and training in acupuncture. Most states require acupuncturists to obtain a license to practice, though states vary in their licensing requirements. Make sure your practitioner is licensed if they are practicing in a state that requires this. Also make sure to ask your practitioner if she or he uses single-use, sterile, and disposable needles that are thrown away after each patient.

Exercise: Tai Chi

A 2010 study published in the *American Journal of Chinese Medicine* from the department of kinesiology at Louisiana State University showed that long-term tai chi practice increases the nerves' ability and speed in sending signals back to the brain and spinal cord. Gentle movement exercises can reawaken the connections between muscles in the body and between the muscles and the mind. Since tai chi and qigong emphasize focused attention on movement, postural alignment, and controlled breathing, you can learn to perform daily tasks with less pain and experience more comfort overall. This is a simple tai chi move that you can perform in the comfort of your home.

1. Stand firmly on the ground with your feet up to shoulder-width apart. Keep your knees slightly bent and your arms relaxed at the sides.

2. Place your right palm on your lower stomach, about two inches below your navel. Push in lightly.

3. Gently put pressure on your stomach as you take a breath in through your nose and exhale through your mouth.

4. Start focusing on relaxing each body part by doing a mental scan from one body part to another.

5. You might notice your body start to sway a bit, which is normal. If this happens, you need to root yourself. Imagine that your feet are the roots of a tree. Focus on staying balanced and firm, as though you are part

Continued >

Exercise: Tai Chi continued

of the ground. Imagine your limbs are the branches, gently and slowly swaying back and forth.

6. Bring your arms up from the side and breathe in. Then slowly bring them down as you breathe out. The movement should be slow and intentional. Try to find a good, comfortable rhythm as you breathe. Make sure your wrists are relaxed.

7. Do the same movement except bring your arms in front of your chest. Bring them down.

8. With your right foot, step out at a 45-degree angle. Use your arms to push out. Imagine there are waves moving in and you're pushing the water out with your arms.

Tip: You can find a link in the Resources on page 199 to see how this is done. For more instructions, it is best to join a class so you can learn more techniques. To see significant results, commit to practicing tai chi three to four times a week.

Nutritional Therapy: Super Anti-Inflammatory Juice

Drinking a fresh green juice that is made from mostly vegetables (and some fruit) is a wonderful way to absorb a lot of nutrients in an efficient manner. It's also an important piece of an effective anti-inflammatory diet plan, which can aid in reducing pain in the body.

You can use a variety of vegetables such as kale, celery, cucumbers, lettuce, spinach, carrot, and beets. Try including apples or pears to sweeten it.

Add a touch of ginger or turmeric for their powerful anti-inflammatory and antioxidant effects. Ginger can offer relief from nerve pain and help with digestion as well.

Super Anti-Inflammatory Juice
- 1-inch knob of ginger (or turmeric)
- 2 cups cherries, pitted
- 1 large cucumber
- 1 small apple, cored and sliced
- 3 stalks celery

1. Place the ginger or turmeric, cherries, cucumber, and apple in a juicer.
2. Place the celery in the juicer last so it can push any soft ingredients through.
3. Drink immediately for best results.

Tip: You can double the recipe and store the remainder of juice in a tightly covered glass container; it will keep in the refrigerator for up to 2 days. If you don't have cherries, you can buy 100% cherry juice from the supermarket and add about ¼ cup to the juice.

OSTEOPOROSIS

Osteoporosis is a condition that affects the skeletal system in which large porous areas develop inside the bone, causing weakened bone structure and a decrease in bone mass. According to the National Institutes of Health Osteoporosis and Related Bone Diseases National Resources Center, "Up to 90 percent of peak bone mass is acquired by age 18 in girls and by age 20 in boys." The amount of bone tissue (bone mass) in your skeleton continues to grow but reaches a maximum in your late 20s. That means prevention of osteoporosis should start as early as possible.

Low bone mass increases the risk of developing osteoporosis. Some of the risk factors that affect bone mass include diet, sex, hormonal factors, exercise, and lifestyle activities. Bones are living organisms, and they're constantly building and breaking down. Women begin to break down slightly faster than they typically rebuild postmenopause, when estrogen levels start to decline. That's why it's important to provide your body with bone-building nutrients such as calcium, magnesium, vitamins D_2, D_3, C, boron, and trace minerals. While supplements can be helpful, vitamins don't get absorbed into the body as well as food sources do. Focus on eating more dark leafy greens, eggs, oily fish, and almonds. Consider drinking herbal infusions, which are highly concentrated and full of beneficial nutrients.

Nutritional Therapy: Bone-Building Nourishing Bowl

Nourishing bowls are quick and easy to make. They contain a perfect balance of vitamins and essential minerals that support your bones. This recipe is very versatile. You can rotate the dark green leafy vegetables such as broccoli, baby kale, and sprouts to suit your tastes. Also, sesame seeds are super high in calcium as an added benefit.

- 1 egg
- 1 small carrot
- ½ avocado
- ½ cup cooked brown rice or quinoa
- 1 cup dark leafy vegetables
- ½ cup blueberries
- 1 teaspoon sesame seeds
- 1 teaspoon pumpkin seeds
- 1 tablespoon pesto
- ½ lemon
- 1 tablespoon extra-virgin olive oil or avocado oil

1. Place the egg in a pot and add cold water until the whole egg is covered and there's an additional 1 inch of water on top.
2. Bring the water to a boil over medium-high heat, then cover.

Continued >

Nutritional Therapy: Bone-Building Nourishing Bowl continued

3. Remove from the heat and set aside for 8 to 10 minutes, then drain and place the egg in a bowl of cold water to cool. Once cooled, remove and peel the egg.

4. Grate the carrot and slice the avocado.

5. Place the cooked rice at the bottom of a medium-size bowl. On top, place the egg, green vegetables, carrot, avocado, blueberries, sesame seeds, pumpkin seeds, and pesto.

6. Squeeze the lemon over the bowl and finish with a drizzle of olive oil.

Herbs: Bone-Repairing Tea

A study from *Nutrition Research* shows that green tea contains polyphenols that support protection against osteoporosis. Rooibos is another bone-benefiting tea that originates from South Africa. The tea is rich in antioxidants that reduce inflammation and flavonoids that promote mineral levels for the bone cells. In addition, rooibos tea contains minerals such as calcium and magnesium.

1. Add 1 tablespoon of loose-leaf green tea or rooibos tea (option: mix ½ tablespoon of each) to a teapot.

2. Boil 1 cup of water, and let it cool for 1 minute. The water should be between 180 and 190 degrees Fahrenheit (82 to 89 degrees Celsius).

3. Pour the hot water in the teapot and steep for 3 minutes.

4. Drink immediately.

Exercise: Qigong—Beginner's Gentle Sway

Regular exercise can slow the progress of many degenerative bone disorders. It is recommended that you do a combination of weight-bearing exercises, like a daily 30-minute walk or light weight training, and flexibility exercises such as tai chi or qigong. Qigong (pronounced "chee-gung") is a 5,000-year-old system of Chinese energy exercises that benefits the mind, body, and spirit. This ancient practice consists of movements, breathing techniques, and meditation. It's designed to develop and improve the circulation of qi, or vital life force.

You can practice qigong by enrolling in a class at your local exercise studio or signing up for an online course such as Chi Center, which is taught by Master Mingtong Gu. According to Master Gu, the best time to do qigong is during the beginning of the day and at the end of the day. Try this beginner's qigong exercise.

1. Stand with both feet wide apart and planted firmly on the ground.

Continued >

Exercise: Qigong—Beginner's Gentle Sway continued

2. Put both hands on your waist and slowly move your upper body to the right. Keeping your head lowered, move your body to the left side and slowly return to the center.

3. Repeat this motion beginning in the opposite direction.

PSORIASIS

Psoriasis is a skin condition that can present in different ways on various parts of the body. Depending on the type, physical symptoms can involve red skin with white scaly patches or small pink spots. Sometimes the patches can feel itchy or have a burning sensation. Unfortunately, there is no known cure for psoriasis. However, there are remedies to provide relief from the itchy and painful symptoms.

Since psoriasis is a chronic inflammatory disease of the skin, joints, and nails, it is imperative that you approach this holistically by addressing the possible underlying issues, which may include diabetes, heart disease, and depression. There are a ton of ways you can manage the superficial symptoms by addressing the inflammation. Consuming vitamin D and a high-quality fish oil supplement and using aloe vera are a few things that can prevent the symptoms from getting worse. You should also avoid chemicals from harsh soaps that can dry out your skin. Keep your skin hydrated, but also keep your body hydrated from the inside out by drinking a lot of water.

Hydrotherapy: Oatmeal and Salt Bath

Oatmeal baths traditionally have been used to soothe dry, itchy, inflamed skin. A study in the *International Journal of Dermatology* shows that bathing in a Dead Sea salt solution improved skin barrier function and reduced skin roughness and inflammation. These salts are mineral salts that have been extracted from the Dead Sea located between Israel and Jordan in southwestern Asia. They contain beneficial minerals such as magnesium, potassium, sodium, and calcium. The high magnesium content provides relief for the skin.

Essential oils are optional, but tea tree oil can enhance the experience due to its anti-inflammatory properties. This can be helpful if you have psoriasis symptoms on your scalp. Simply add about five drops to your shampoo and massage your scalp. For mild psoriasis conditions, taking this bath three times a week is enough. For more severe conditions, you can take this bath once a day.

- 2 cups Dead Sea salt
- ½ cup natural colloidal oatmeal
- Tea tree oil (optional)

1. Fill a bathtub with warm water.
2. Dissolve the salt while the water is running.
3. Add the oatmeal and tea tree oil (if using).
4. Soak for 20 minutes.

5. While your skin is still damp, apply a moisturizer such as extra-virgin coconut oil or olive oil.

Tip: You can grind up oatmeal to a fine powder or buy pre-ground colloidal oatmeal to save time. To make oat flour, simply blend rolled oats in a high-speed blender until powdery soft. If you can't find Dead Sea salt, you can also use Epsom salt.

Herb: Chai Tonic Tea

Herbal teas like chai, when taken regularly, are one of the best ways to relieve inflammation. Combine a diet rich in anti-inflammatory foods with a nourishing cup of chai tea. To really experience the tea at a therapeutic level, consider drinking chai tea as a tonic—a preparation of herbs that supports health and well-being.

- 1 cup coconut milk
- 1 teaspoon turmeric powder
- ½ teaspoon cinnamon
- ¼ teaspoon ground ginger
- Pinch pink pepper
- ½ teaspoon coconut oil
- ¼ teaspoon vanilla extract
- ½ to 1 teaspoon raw honey, to taste

Continued >

Herb: Chai Tonic Tea continued

1. Heat the coconut milk in a small pot over low heat.

2. Add the turmeric, cinnamon, ginger, pepper, coconut oil, and vanilla.

3. Simmer for 20 minutes, being careful not to bring to a boil.

4. Pour into a mug, and strain out the spices if you prefer.

5. Add honey to taste.

Tip: This is very creamy chai. You can replace some of the milk with water if you prefer.

Essential Oil and Herb: Aloe Vera and Tea Tree Oil Paste

Aloe vera is a succulent plant that is used for its soothing properties. The gel that contains the healing compounds includes essential amino acids, antioxidants, fatty acids, and minerals. It's also antimicrobial, antiviral, antifungal, and antibacterial. Aloe vera has natural soothing properties that help deal with redness and scaling. It naturally contains many active constituents including salicylic acid, which helps promote skin turnover. It also contains vitamins A, C, and E to help nourish the skin.

Adding tea tree oil to aloe vera makes it an even more potent remedy. Tea tree oil is a broad-spectrum antimicrobial agent that can help heal the skin and prevent infections, if your skin has cracks.

- 1 (2-foot) fresh aloe leaf (or ½ cup pure aloe vera gel)
- ¼ cup coconut oil
- 10 drops tea tree essential oil

1. Use a small knife to carefully slice open the aloe leaf. Scoop the clear gel out with a spoon and put it in a blender.

2. Add the coconut oil.

3. Blend for 30 to 60 seconds until combined.

4. Put the mixture in a glass container. Add the tea tree oil.

5. Scoop out about 1 tablespoon and apply to skin. Use more if needed. Let it sit for 20 minutes and rinse with water and mild soap. If you use it on your scalp, wash off with a mild shampoo.

6. Store the remainder in the refrigerator.

STRESS

Stressful experiences are a normal part of life, and the stress response is a survival mechanism that primes us to respond to threats. Some stress is positive, such as acute stress. But when a stressor is negative and can't be fought off or avoided or when the experience of stress becomes chronic, our biological responses to stress can impair our physical and mental health. Fortunately, there are many holistic tools to help combat the negative effects of stress in healthy ways.

Emotional Freedom Techniques

Tapping, also known as the Emotional Freedom Technique (EFT), is a technique that combines ancient Chinese acupressure and modern psychology. You use your fingers to lightly tap specific acupressure points on the face and upper body to help relieve tension and stress. Best of all, you can do this to yourself anywhere, at any time. Drawing from the concept that we all have energy that flows through our bodies on pathways called meridians, tapping on these meridian points can break up blockages. We can lower the cortisol levels that lead to negative emotions.

1. Take a deep breath. On a scale of 1 to 10, how stressed are you? Get clear on that number in your head.

2. Curl your left hand and begin by tapping under that hand. As you tap on the different points, say the sentences in quotation marks aloud. "Even though I am totally stressed out, I deeply and completely accept myself."

3. Tap on the top of your eyebrows. "This stress has been really blocking me."

4. Tap on the side of the eye. "This stress has been holding me back in every area of my life."

5. Tap under the eye. "All this stress."

6. Tap under your nose. "All this stress is holding me back."

7. Tap your chin. "All this stress is making me feel extremely uncomfortable."

8. Tap your collarbone. "All this stress is making me feel like I can't move forward with my life."

9. Tap your underarm. "All this stress is making me feel sick."

10. Tap the top of your head. "This stress is overwhelming me."

Continued >

REMEDIES

11. Repeat this sequence.

12. Take a deep breath. Now ask yourself on a scale of 1 to 10, how stressed are you? Repeat until you feel a sense of relief.

Tip: You can see how this technique is done in Gabrielle Bernstein's video listed in the Resources.

Herbs: Bulletproof Mushroom Latte

This cozy mushroom latte may be your next replacement for coffee in the morning. Mushrooms have long been touted for their health benefits. They're loaded with vitamins, minerals, and have healing properties. The superstar ingredients in this medicinal latte are reishi and chaga. Reishi mushrooms have been used for thousands of years by Taoist monks to support the immune system and reduce stress and anxiety. They have been thought to open up the crown chakra, which is located at the top of your forehead. Chaga mushrooms contain high amounts of the antioxidant enzyme superoxide dismutase, which neutralizes free radicals in the body. They also help the body deal with everyday stress. Drinking mushroom lattes can increase your resilience to the damaging effects of chronic stress and restore balance to your body.

- 1 cup unsweetened cashew or coconut milk
- ½ teaspoon reishi mushroom powder
- ½ teaspoon chaga mushroom powder
- ½ teaspoon maca powder
- ¼ teaspoon cinnamon
- 1 tablespoon cacao powder
- 2 teaspoons honey or maple syrup
- 1 teaspoon coconut oil or ghee

1. Place all ingredients in a small saucepan and gently warm over medium heat until they come to a simmer. Gently stir.

2. Carefully transfer the hot liquid to a high-speed blender and blend on high for 30 seconds, or until the latte is frothy. If you don't have a blender, simply whisk vigorously until it's creamy.

3. Pour into a mug and enjoy!

Meditation: Kundalini Meditation for Stress Relief

Kundalini is the practice of honoring the teacher within you. It teaches you to have a connection with your nervous system. Kundalini meditation is practiced by chanting and doing breath work, which has been known to relieve stress

Continued >

REMEDIES

and anxiety. The following meditation practice helps clear emotional tension and stress.

1. Sit in any cross-legged posture. Elongate your spine. Close your eyes.

2. Each kundalini practice begins with the opening chant *Ong Namo Guru Dev Namo,* which means "I bow to the teacher within."

3. Rub your hands together and close your eyes. Chant the phrase from step 2 three times. Take a deep breath in between each chant.

4. Put your hands on each of your knees. Inhale and hold your breath. Hold your breath as you flex your spine. Using the leverage of your hands on your knees, move your spine and chest in a snake-like motion, forward and backward, as you hold your breath. Move at a comfortable rhythm.

5. Exhale as you come to the center and stop rocking your spine.

6. End the meditation by inhaling and holding your breath for as long as you feel comfortable.

7. Do this for up to 20 minutes whenever you feel stressed.

THYROID IMBALANCE

Thyroid disorders are conditions that affect the thyroid gland and its metabolic functions. There are typically two kinds of conditions—hyperthyroidism and hypothyroidism. Symptoms that occur in hyperthyroidism include weight loss, fatigue, mood swings, and menstrual inconsistency. Symptoms in hypothyroidism include weight gain, cold intolerance, hair loss, puffy face, depression, body aches, stiff muscles, and irregular menstrual cycles. Effective holistic remedies usually include supporting the digestive system, adrenal glands, and the liver's detoxification pathways. Lifestyle choices such as stress management, self-care, and diet are also very important in managing thyroid health.

Nutrition Therapy: Digestive Bitters

If you're going to balance your thyroid, it's critical to first heal your gut. Over 70 percent of your immune system resides in your gut, commonly referred to as gut-associated lymphoid tissue. Digestive problems such as sluggish intestinal mobility and constipation have been linked to hypothyroidism. Digestive bitters are an infusion of bitter botanicals that include herbs, flowers, fruit, seeds,

Continued >

REMEDIES

---

and bark. They can ramp up digestive function, improving digestion and absorption of foods.

Bitters also help increase digestive juices, called hydrochloric acid (HCl), in the stomach. This is necessary for the breakdown of food and absorption of essential nutrients such as iron. Since iron is used to make thyroid hormones, having low HCl can lead to thyroid problems. Bitters also increase the detoxification process in the liver and have a positive effect on stress due to the gut-brain connection. You can buy digestive bitters that have a combination of herbs, or you can incorporate more plant-based foods with bitter compounds including kale, Brussels sprouts, grapefruit, arugula, dandelion, and watercress. Buy digestive bitters from your local health food store, ideally a blend that contains dandelion, burdock root, artichoke leaf, wormwood, and chamomile.

Take one full dropper (about ¼ teaspoon) of the bitters on your tongue and swallow. You can take it before a meal up to five times a day to help with digestion.

Detoxification: Liver Detox Smoothie

When it comes to supporting your thyroid, most people probably focus on healing only that organ. The liver has over 500 functions and one of them is to convert the

T4 hormone to the active T3 hormone. So if your liver is impaired, your body may not have sufficient levels of active T3, which is responsible for metabolism, hair growth, and energy.

The liver is our body's primary detoxification organ. To support the detox pathways, the liver needs vitamins and nutrients such as B vitamins, glutathione, and folate. When too many toxins accumulate, factored with possible exposure to heavy metals, you're at risk for having an overburdened liver. You can support your liver by eating nutrient-dense foods, such as this smoothie recipe.

Spirulina and chlorella can bind to and remove heavy metals and other toxins that might otherwise tax your liver. Lab studies show that chlorella can absorb 40 percent of heavy metals in a test solution within seven days, while animal studies show that chlorella helps remove toxins like mercury from the body. Chlorella also contains several nutrients with antioxidant properties, including vitamin C, chlorophyll, beta-carotene, lutein, and lycopene. Brazil nuts contain selenium, which helps prevent oxidative damage to your thyroid.

- ½ lemon, juiced
- 1 orange, peeled
- 1 cup wild blueberries
- 1 banana, peeled

Continued >

Detoxification: Liver Detox Smoothie continued

- 1 teaspoon spirulina
- 1 tablespoon chlorella
- 1 tablespoon chia seeds
- 1 pinch cinnamon
- 2 cups filtered water or nut milk of choice
- 2 Brazil nuts
- Ice (optional)

1. Combine all the ingredients in a high-speed blender.
2. Drink and enjoy once a day.

Herb: Matcha Zen Latte

Stress can have a negative effect on your thyroid function. A common example of chronic stress is adrenal fatigue, which occurs when your adrenal glands are unable to keep up with physiological needs. One way to combat this is to reduce coffee consumption. Replace it with a matcha green tea latte, which contains L-theanine that reduces cortisol and helps you feel calmer. Try adding adaptogenic herbs to your drinks. Adaptogens have been shown to decrease levels of cortisol, a stress hormone secreted when our body experiences stress. Ashwagandha, an adaptogenic herb in Ayurveda, is often used to support thyroid health by helping the body adapt to daily stress.

Sip on this latte and do some deep breathing or meditation in the morning. Your thyroid and adrenals will thank you.

- ½ to 1 teaspoon organic matcha green tea powder
- ½ cup hot water (just below boiling)
- ½ to 1 cup coconut milk (oat milk and almond milk are great alternatives)
- 1 heaping tablespoon of coconut cream or collagen powder (honey, maple syrup, or yacon syrup)

1. For the best texture, whisk the matcha green tea powder with ½ cup of hot water using a bamboo whisk in a small round bowl. This breaks up any clumps, and will make the latte taste creamier.

2. Pour the matcha mixture into your favorite mug. Whisk with a bamboo whisk until dissolved.

3. Heat the coconut milk on the stovetop or in a frothing pitcher.

4. Pour the milk into your mug and enjoy immediately.

Tip: If you don't have a bamboo whisk, use a spoon or blend the latte in a blender for the creamiest texture.

URINARY TRACT INFECTIONS

Urinary tract infections (UTIs) are very common, especially in women, because they have a shorter urethra, the tube that connects to the urinary bladder where bacteria can easily enter. The infection may occur in any part of the urinary system but most commonly occurs in the bladder. UTIs are infections that are caused by the overgrowth of bacteria in the urinary system, which can be very painful.

While antibiotics are effective for treating complicated cases of UTI, the body can restore minor symptoms on its own without the help of antibiotics. In fact, there is a trade-off for overusing antibiotics, especially if you have recurrent UTIs. The overuse of antibiotics can cause bacteria resistance.

In addition to the remedies provided in this section, remember to drink plenty of water throughout the day to flush the bacteria from your system. Avoid all sugar and dairy and drink lots of fluid. Drinking cranberry juice can also help prevent recurrent UTIs if you experience symptoms. However, if you experience serious symptoms, especially for recurrent UTIs, such as fevers, chills, or extreme pain, see a doctor immediately. When in doubt, make an appointment with your doctor.

Probiotics: Kombucha Lemonade

One of the key remedies for UTIs is to double up on your probiotics. A study published in the *Turkish Journal of Urology* shows that taking probiotics that contain the lactobacillus species can help alleviate the symptoms of UTI by preventing the adherence, growth, and colonization of bacteria.

In addition to taking a high-quality probiotic supplement, you can also consume fermented tea or fermented foods to help restore your body's natural flora and allow the healthy bacteria to multiply. Kombucha is a delicious and refreshing fermented green or black tea that contains both probiotics and antioxidants. Make sure you choose one that has a low amount of sugar, preferably no more than 5 grams. When you feel the UTI symptoms creeping up, immediately start doubling up your dose of probiotic supplements, in addition to drinking this kombucha lemonade. If you have a powdered probiotic supplement, feel free to mix in one serving.

- 1 (16- to 24-ounce) bottle premade kombucha
- 1 lemon
- Ice

1. Pour the entire contents of the kombucha bottle into a large glass.
2. Cut the lemon and squeeze all the juice into the glass.
3. Add ice and drink immediately.

Nutritional Therapy: Cranberry and Aloe Vera Spa Water

Drink 100 percent pure cranberry juice (no sugar added) diluted with water to flush out the kidneys and bladder. An article from *Clinics* (São Paulo) shows that cranberry has vitamin C, antioxidants, and polyphenols that function as a natural defense mechanism against bacteria. It's more effective as a preventive measure than a cure for UTI, although it does benefit you by making you urinate more frequently, which can decrease bacterial growth and keep you hydrated.

- 4 to 5 mint leaves
- ½ cucumber
- Ice
- ½ cup pure cranberry juice concentrate
- 1 cup aloe vera juice
- 2 cups filtered water

1. Bruise the mint leaves by slapping them between your palms to release the natural oils, and place the leaves in a large mason jar.

2. Cut the cucumber into thin slices and add to the jar.

3. Add ice.

4. Fill the jar with the cranberry juice, aloe vera juice, and water, and gently stir with a straw or spoon.

5. Drink throughout the day.

Tip: You can also take cranberry extract capsules (about 400 milligrams) with D-mannose (1000 milligrams), a nondigestible sugar that attaches to bacteria and flushes them out when you urinate.

Homeopathic Remedy: Cantharis 30C

For more acute UTI symptoms, you can try homeopathic remedies. Homeopathic remedies are derived from different natural substances. Due to the high level of dilution (not as concentrated as herbs), homeopathy is considered safe and nontoxic.

If you feel a burning sensation during urination, it's helpful to use Cantharis 30C, which is a homeopathic formula. Cantharis 30C is an effective and commonly used remedy for UTI because it can relieve symptoms such as a burning sensation and decreased urine flow. You can buy this formula at a health food store, a pharmacy such as Walgreens or CVS, or online. Make sure you buy from a reputable brand such as Boiron or Hyland's.

Put five pellets under the tongue, three times a day, until your symptoms improve.

PARTING WORDS

My hope is that after reading this book, you will be empowered to take responsibility for and control of your own health. You can reclaim the self-healing powers inside of you as you heal with all that nature has to offer. *You* are your own healer. Your body is the true healer.

There is a powerful connection between your body and mind. You can change your beliefs and attitudes and their effects on your body and mind. Learn to listen to your body and hear what it's saying and what it needs.

With the right supporting health-care team, environment, techniques, and ancient wisdom from this book, your body will innately begin to achieve balance toward optimal health. I truly hope you are able to find a team of supportive practitioners in the holistic field to support you through this transformative journey.

Good luck and embrace the joy in your healing journey!

RESOURCES

Preparation is key. Having the remedies and tools you need in your home makes it less stressful when an ailment shows up. It is best to purchase ingredients that are organic and/or expeller pressed. When it comes to buying herbs, quality is important. Always purchase your herbs from a trusted source. Make sure they are USDA-certified organic and wild-crafted. Your holistic and natural medicine will only be as good as the quality of the herbs and how they were grown.

RECOMMENDED PLACES TO SHOP

The following is a list of places where you can buy the ingredients for the remedies:

Health food stores (Sprouts, Whole Foods, etc.)
Local farmers' markets (fresh whole foods, raw honey)
Mountain Rose Herbs (herbs, tea)
doTERRA (essential oils)
Young Living (essential oils)
Thrive Market (affordable online health food store)
Frontier Co-op (herbs)
Original Bach Flower Remedies (flower essences)

RECOMMENDED READING

Want to read more about holistic practices? Try the following books.

Adaptogens: Herbs for Strength, Stamina, and Stress Relief by David Winston

Ayurveda Lifestyle Wisdom by Acharya Shunya

Clean Skin From Within by Dr. Trevor Cates

Essential Oils for Healing by Vannoy Gentles Fite

Flowerevolution by Katie Hess

Foods That Fight Pain by Dr. Neal Barnard

Manual for Self-Hypnosis by Dr. D. Corydon Hammond

Secrets of Self-Healing by Dr. Maoshing Ni

The Alternative Health & Medicine Encyclopedia by James Marti

The Bach Flower Remedies by Dr. Edward Bach

The Encyclopedia of Bach Flower Therapy by Mechthild Scheffer

The End of Diabetes by Dr. Joel Fuhrman

The Essential Oils Complete Reference Guide by KG Stiles

The Magnesium Miracle by Dr. Carolyn Dean

The Reiki Manual by Penelope Quest

RECOMMENDED VIDEOS

The following are some instructional videos that can help you learn how to do some of the exercises in this book.

ABHYANGA MASSAGE

YouTube.com/watch?v=_HQLsfZh5js&t=4s

COBRA POSE

YouTube.com/watch?v=XU0wJ0OTopU

EFT TAPPING TO REDUCE ANXIETY AND STRESS (GABRIELLE BERNSTEIN)

YouTube.com/watch?v=9UiLZGCtSzM

REBOUNDING

YouTube.com/watch?v=GvBPy3Vxl50

TAI CHI

YouTube.com/watch?v=cEOS2zoyQw4

ONLINE RESOURCES FOR FURTHER READING

Acupressure.com

AHHA.org

AthreyaAyurveda.com

Ayurveda.com

AyurvedaNama.org

BachFlower.com

Chopra.com

DoYogaWithMe.com

DrWeil.com

FoundationforPN.org

HealingTouchProgram.com

IARP.org

KundaliniYoga.org

Mindful.org/How-to-Meditate

Mindworks.org

MeghanTelpner.com

NCCIH.NIH.gov

QigongInstitute.org

Reiki.org

TCMWorld.org

TheHerbalAcademy.com

TM.org

YogaBasics.com

YogaInternational.com

YogaJournal.com

REFERENCES

Akgül, Turgay, and Tolga Karakan. "The Role of Probiotics in Women with Recurrent Urinary Tract Infections." *Turkish Journal of Urology* 44, no. 5 (September 2018): 377–83. doi .org/10.5152/tud.2018.48742.

Alda, Marta, Marta Puebla-Guedea, Baltasar Rodero, Marcelo Demarzo, Jesus Montero-Marin, Miquel Roca, and Javier Garcia-Campayo. "Zen Meditation, Length of Telomeres, and the Role of Experiential Avoidance and Compassion." *Mindfulness* (2016) 7: 651–59. doi.org/10.1007 /s12671-016-0500-5.

Ali, Babar, Naser Ali Al-Wabel, Saiba Shams, Aftab Ahamad, Shah Alam Khan, and Firoz Anwar. "Essential Oils Used in Aromatherapy: A Systemic Review." *Asian Pacific Journal of Tropical Biomedicine* 5, no. 8 (2015): 601–11. doi.org/10.1016 /j.apjtb.2015.05.007.

Alirezaei, Mehrdad, Christopher C. Kemball, Claudia T. Flynn, Malcolm R. Wood, J. Lindsay Whitton, and William B. Kiosses. "Short-Term Fasting Induces Profound Neuronal Autophagy." *Autophagy* 6, no. 6 (2010): 702–10. doi.org/10.4161 /auto.6.6.12376.

American Academy of Dermatology. "Acne: Who Gets and Causes." aad.org. aad.org/public/diseases/acne/causes/acne -causes (accessed April 19, 2020).

American Lung Association. "Five Ways You Might Be Breathing Wrong." Lung.org. lung.org/blog/you-might-be -breathing-wrong (accessed March 15, 2020).

Astin, J.A., S. L. Shapiro, D. M. Eisenberg, K. L. Forys. "Mind-body medicine: state of the science, implications for practice." *The Journal of the American Board of Family Practice* (2003) Mar–Apr; 16(2):131–47. doi.org/10.3122/jabfm.16.2.131.

Aziz, Zoriah, Su Yuen Wong, and Nyuk Jet Chong. "Effects of *Hibiscus sabdariffa* L. on Serum Lipids: A Systematic Review and Meta-analysis." *Journal of Ethnopharmacology* 150, no. 2 (November 2013): 442–50. doi.org/10.1016/j.jep.2013.09.042.

Barnard, Neal D. *Foods That Fight Pain: Revolutionary New Strategies for Maximum Pain Relief*. 1st Edition. New York: Harmony Books, 1998.

Benson, Herbert. *Beyond the Relaxation Response: The Stress-Reduction Program That Has Helped Millions of Americans*. Reprint Edition. New York City: Berkley, 1985.

Burden, B., and M. S. Herron. "The Increasing Use of Reiki as a Complementary Therapy in Specialist Palliative Care." *International Journal of Palliative Nursing* (2005) 11, no. 5: 248–53.

Cates, Trevor. "Clean Skin from Within: The Spa Doctor's Two-Week Program to Glowing, Naturally Youthful Skin." Beverly: Fair Winds Press, 2017.

China Education Center. "Introduction to Traditional Chinese Medicine." Accessed March 3, 2020. chinaeducenter.com/en /cedu/tcm.php.

Choonhakarn, C., P. Busaracome, B. Sripanidkulchai, and P. Sarakarn. "A Prospective, Randomized Clinical Trial Comparing Topical Aloe Vera with 0.1% Triamcinolone Acetonide in Mild to Moderate Plaque Psoriasis." *Journal of European Academy Dermatology Venereology* (2010) 24, no. 2: 168–72. doi.org/10.1111/j.1468-3083.2009.03377.x PMid:19686327.

Clarke, T. C., P. M. Barnes, L. I. Black, B. J. Stussman, R. L. Nahin. "Use of yoga, meditation, and chiropractors among U.S. adults aged 18 and older." NCHS Data Brief, no 325. Hyattsville, MD: National Center for Health Statistics. 2018.

Coles, Leah T., and Peter M. Clifton. "Effect of Beetroot Juice on Lowering Blood Pressure in Free-Living, Disease-Free Adults: A Randomized, Placebo-Controlled Trial." *Nutrition Journal* (2012). doi.org/10.1186/1475-2891-11-106.

Davidson, Richard J., and Antoine Lutz. "Buddha's Brain: Neuroplasticity and Meditation." *IEEE Signal Processing Magazine* (2008) Jan 1; 25(1): 176–174.

De Cabo, Rafael, and Mark P. Mattson. "Effects of Intermittent Fasting on Health, Aging, and Disease." *New England Journal of Medicine* 381, no. 26 (2019): 2541–51. doi.org/10.1056 /NEJMra1905136.

Diane L., C-Y. Oliver Chen, Edward Saltzman, and Jeffrey B. Blumberg. "*Hibiscus sabdariffa* L. Tea (Tisane) Lowers Blood Pressure in Pre-hypertensive and Mildly Hypertensive Adults." *The Journal of Nutrition* (2009). doi.org/10.3945 /jn.109.115097.

Eden, Donna, and David Feinstein. *Energy Medicine: Balancing Your Body's Energies for Optimal Health, Joy, and Vitality*. New York City: TarcherPerigee, 2008.

Ernst, E. "Obstacles to Research in Complementary and Alternative Medicine." *Medical Journal of Australia* 179, no. 6 (2003): 279–80.

Fuhrman, Joel, and Michael Singer. "Improved Cardiovascular Parameter with a Nutrient-Dense, Plant-Rich Diet-Style: A Patient Survey with Illustrative Cases." *American Journal of Lifestyle Medicine* (2015). doi.org/10.1177/1559827615611024.

Future Market Insights. "Herbal Medicinal Products Market." FutureMarketInsights.com. futuremarketinsights.com/reports /herbal-medicinal-products-market (accessed April 19, 2020).

Gröber, Uwe, Tanja Werner, Jürgen Vormann, and Klaus Kisters. "Myth or Reality—Transdermal Magnesium?" *Nutrients* 9, no. 8 (2017): 813. doi.org/10.3390/nu9080813.

Harvard T. H. Chan School of Public Health. "Processed Foods and Health." *The Nutrition Source*. Accessed March 2, 2020. hsph.harvard.edu/nutritionsource/processed-foods.

Hisano, Marcelo, Homero Bruschini, Antonio Carlos Nicodemo, and Miguel Srougi. "Cranberries and lower urinary tract infection prevention." *Clinics* (2012) Jun; 67(6): 661–667. doi.org/10.6061/clinics/2012(06)18.

Jaewon, Wenzhen Duan, Jeffrey M. Long, Donald K. Ingram, and Mark P. Mattson. "Dietary Restriction Increases the Number of Newly Generated Neural Cells, and Induces BDNF Expression, in the Dentate Gyrus of Rats." *International Journal of Molecular Sciences* 15, no. 2 (2000): 99–108. doi.org/10.1385/JMN:15:2:99.

Jahnke, Roger, Linda Larkey, PhD, Carol Rogers, Jennifer Etnier, and Fang Lin. "A Comprehensive Review of Health Benefits of Qigong and Tai Chi." *American Journal of Health Promotion* (2010) Jul-Aug; 24(6): e1–e25. doi/org/10.4278/ajhp.081013-LIT-248.

Jin, Hee-Kyung, Tae-Yeon Hwang, and Sung-Hyoun Cho. "Effect of Electrical Stimulation on Blood Flow Velocity and Vessel Size." *Open Medicine Institute.* 12, no. 1 (2017). doi.org/10.1515/med-2017-0002.

Kang, Sun, Le Wang, Qingping Ma, Qiaoyun Cui, Qianru Lv, Wenzheng Zhang, and Xinghui Li. "Association between Tea Consumption and Osteoporosis." *Medicine Baltimore* 96, no. 49 (December 2017). doi.org/10.1097/MD.0000000000009034.

Ko, Chun Hay, Kit Man Lau, Wing Yee Choy, Ping Chung Leung. "Effects of Tea Catechins, Epigallocatechin, Gallocatechin, and

Gallocatechin Gallate, on Bone Metabolism." J. Agric. Food Chem. August (2009): 57 (16), pp 7293-7297. doi.org/10.1021/jf901545u.

Koithan, Mary. "Introducing Complementary and Alternative Therapies." *Journal of Nurse Practitioners* (2009) 5, no. 1 (January 2009): 18–20. doi.org/10.1016/j.nurpra.2008.10.012.

Lake, James, MD. Integrative Mental Health Care: A Therapist's Handbook (Norton Professional Books), 1st Edition. New York: W. W. Norton & Company, 2015.

Lämås, Kristina, Lars Lindholmb, Hans Stenlund, Birgitta Engström, and Catrine Jacobsson. "Effects of Abdominal Massage in Management of Constipation—A Randomized Controlled Trial." *International Journal of Nursing Studies* 46, no. 6 (2009): 759–67. doi.org/10.1016/j.ijnurstu.2009.01.007.

Lee, Jiyeon, Marylin Dodd, Suzanne Dibble, and Donald Abrams. "Review of Acupressure Studies for Chemotherapy-Induced Nausea and Vomiting Control." *Oncology Nursing Forum* 36, no. 5 (November 2008): 529–44. doi.org/10.1016/j.jpainsymman.2007.10.019.

Lete, I., and J. Allue. "The Effectiveness of Ginger in the Prevention of Nausea and Vomiting during Pregnancy and Chemotherapy." *Integrative Medicine Insights* 11 (2016): 11–17. doi.org/10.4137/IMI.S36273.

Ling, Yang, Dan Yang, and Wenlong Shao. "Understanding Vomiting from the Perspective of Traditional Chinese Medicine." *Annals of Palliative Medicine* 1, no. 2 (2012).

Min-sun, Juyoung Lee, Bum-Jin Park, and Yoshifumi Miyazak. "Interaction with Indoor Plants May Reduce Psychological and Physiological Stress by Suppressing Autonomic Nervous System Activity in Young Adults: A Randomized Crossover Study." *Journal of Physiological Anthropology* 34, no. 21 (2015).

Mozaffari-Khosravi, H. "The Effects of Sour Tea (*Hibiscus sabdariffa*) on Hypertension in Patients with Type II Diabetes." *Journal of Human Hypertension* 23 (August 2008): 48–54. doi.org/10.1038/jhh.2008.100.

Nash, L. A., and W. E. Ward. "Comparison of Black, Green and Rooibos Tea on Osteoblast Activity." *Food & Function* 7, no. 2 (February 2016): 1166–75. doi.org/10.1039/c5fo01222h.

NIH Osteoporosis and Related Bone Diseases National Resources Center. "Osteoporosis Overview." NIH.gov. bones.nih.gov/health-info/bone/osteoporosis/overview (accessed March 12, 2020).

Patwardhan, Bhushan, Dnyaneshwar Warude, P. Pushpangadan, and Narendra Bhatt. "Ayurveda and Traditional Chinese Medicine: A Comparative Overview." *Evidence-Based Complementary and Alternative Medicine* 2, no. 4 (2005): 465–73. doi.org/10.1093/ecam/neh140.

Pawluk, William. "Power Tools for Health: How pulsed magnetic fields (PEMFs) help you." Victoria BC: FriesenPress 2017.

Proksch, E., H. P. Nissen, M. Bremgartner, and C. Urquhart. "Bathing in a magnesium-rich Dead Sea salt solution improves skin barrier function, enhances skin hydration, and reduces inflammation in atopic dry skin." *International Journal of Dermatology* (2005) Feb;44(2): 151-7. doi.org /10.1111/j.1365-4632.2005.02079.x.

Sedwick, Caitlin. "Yoshinori Ohsumi: Autophagy from Beginning to End." *Journal of Cell Biology* 197, no. 2 (2012): 164–65. doi.org/10.1083/jcb.1972pi.

Selye, Hans. The Stress of Life. 2nd Edition. New York City: McGraw-Hill, 1978.

Shen, Chwan-Li, James K. Yeh, Jay J. Cao, and Jia-Sheng Wang. "Green Tea and Bone Metabolism." *Nutrition* (2009) 29, no. 7: 437–56. doi.org/10.1016/j.nutres.2009.06.008.

Sinclair, Marybetts. "The Use of Abdominal Massage to Treat Chronic Constipation." *Journal of Bodywork and Movement Therapies* 15, no. 4 (2011): 436–45. doi.org/10.1016 /j.jbmt.2010.07.007.

Sites, Debra S., Nancy T. Johnson, Jacqueline A. Miller, Jennifer Nance, Tara H. Fox, and Rebecca Creech Tart. "Controlled Breathing with or without Peppermint Aromatherapy for Postoperative Nausea and/or Vomiting Symptom Relief: A

Randomized Controlled Trial." *Journal of Paranesthesia Nursing* 29, no. 1 (2014): 12–19. doi.org/10.1016/j.jopan.2013.09.008.

Sleep Foundation. "National Foundation Recommends New Sleep Times." SleepFoundation.org. sleepfoundation.org/press -release/national-sleep-foundation-recommends-new-sleep -times (accessed April 19, 2020).

So, P. S., Y. Jiang, and Y. Qin. "Touch Therapies for Pain Relief in Adults." *Cochrane Database of Systematic Reviews* 4 (2008).

St. Marie, Raymond, and Kellie S. Talebkhah. "Neurological Evidence of a Mind-Body Connection: Mindfulness and Pain Control." *American Journal of Psychiatry* (2018). doi.org /10.1176/appi.ajp-rj.2018.130401.

U.S. Department of Health & Human Services: The National Institutes of Health. Accessed April 24, 2012. nih.gov.

Uvnas-Moberg. Kerstin. *Oxytocin Factor: With a New Foreword: Tapping the Hormone of Calm, Love and Healing.* 2nd Edition. London: Pinter & Martin Ltd, 2011.

Wahabi, H. A., L. A. Alansary, A. H. Al-Sabban, and P. Glasziuo. "The Effectiveness of *Hibiscus sabdariffa* in the Treatment of Hypertension: A Systematic Review." *Phytomedicine* (February 2010): 83–6.

White, Mathew P., Ian Alcock, James Grellier, Benedict W. Wheeler, Terry Hartig, Sara L. Warber, Angie Bone, Michael H. Depledge, and Lora E. Fleming. "Spending at Least

120 Minutes a Week in Nature Is Associated with Good Health and Wellbeing." *Scientific Reports* 9, no. 1 (2019). doi.org /10.1038/s41598-019-44097-3.

Wolsko, Peter M., David M. Eisenberg, Roger B. Davis, and Russell S. Phillips. "Use of Mind-Body Medical Therapies. *Journal of General Internal Medicine* 19, no. 1 (January 2004): 43–50. doi .org/10.1111/j.1525-1497.2004.21019.x.

Woodyard, Catherine. "Exploring the therapeutic effects of yoga and its ability to increase quality of life." *International Journal of Yoga* (2011), Jul-Dec; 4(2): 49–54. doi.org/10.4103 /0973-6131.85485.

Yan, Zhang, Lixing Lao, Haiyan Chen, and Rodrigo Ceballos. "Acupuncture Use among American Adults: What Acupuncture Practitioners Can Learn from National Health Interview Survey 2007?" *Evidence Based Complementary and Alternative Medicine*. (2012) 2012: 710750. doi.org/10.1155/2012 /710750.

Zeidan, Fadel, and David Vago. "Mindfulness Meditation-Based Pain Relief: A Mechanistic Account." *Annals of the New York Academy of Sciences* 1373, no. 1 (June 2016): 114–27. doi.org /10.1111/nyas.13153.

Zhang, Yu-Jie, Ren-You Gan, Sha Li, Yue Zhou, An-Na Li, Dong-Ping Xu, and Hua-Bin Li. "Antioxidant Phytochemicals for the Prevention and Treatment of Chronic Diseases." *Molecules* 20, no. 12 (2015). doi.org/10.3390/molecules201219753.

INDEX

ACKNOWLEDGMENTS

I want to acknowledge my two children, Tyler and Alana, for being my teachers in life. They may be too young to understand and realize it, but they are the real forces that drive my motivation to continue to learn and research everything about health. I want to thank my husband and "night nanny," David, for his loving support and for taking care of our children so I could work on this book.

I am also grateful for my sister, Linda, for constantly reminding me to push through difficult times, providing energizing snacks, and dotting all the i's and crossing all the t's. I would like to thank my parents, Sang and Phong, for their unconditional love and wisdom. I would not be here chasing my dreams if they let fear stop them from stepping on that boat 35 years ago.

I have tremendous gratitude for all my teachers at the Institute for Integrative Nutrition who provided me with the knowledge and foundation for my education. I am also extremely thankful and appreciative of the talented and patient team of editors and designers for all their hard work in creating this book. Without them, everything would still remain in my head and not shared with the world.

ABOUT THE AUTHOR

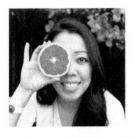 **KIM LAM, AADP, CHHC,** is a holistic health coach and founder of Lettuce Be Healthy, helping clients rediscover their health through her holistic approach, which uniquely combines scientific evidence with intuitive coaching and ancient wisdom. She specializes in educating and empowering busy mothers and corporate women on mindful and intuitive eating, lifestyle, healthy habits, digestive health, and detoxification.

Kim's holistic approach to health and wellness focuses on food nutrition and all aspects of life including sleep, stress, emotions, and eating habits. She obtained her training from the Institute for Integrative Nutrition and graduated as a health coach.

Kim currently lives in Northern California with her husband, two young kids, and two dogs who keep her on her toes. She enjoys cooking and developing healthy recipes, running half marathons, yoga, traveling, and spending time in the woods.

CPSIA information can be obtained
at www.ICGtesting.com
Printed in the USA
BVHW020322200620
581764BV00022B/184

9 781647 396084